STEP-BY-STEP
YOGA
FOR STRESS RELIEF

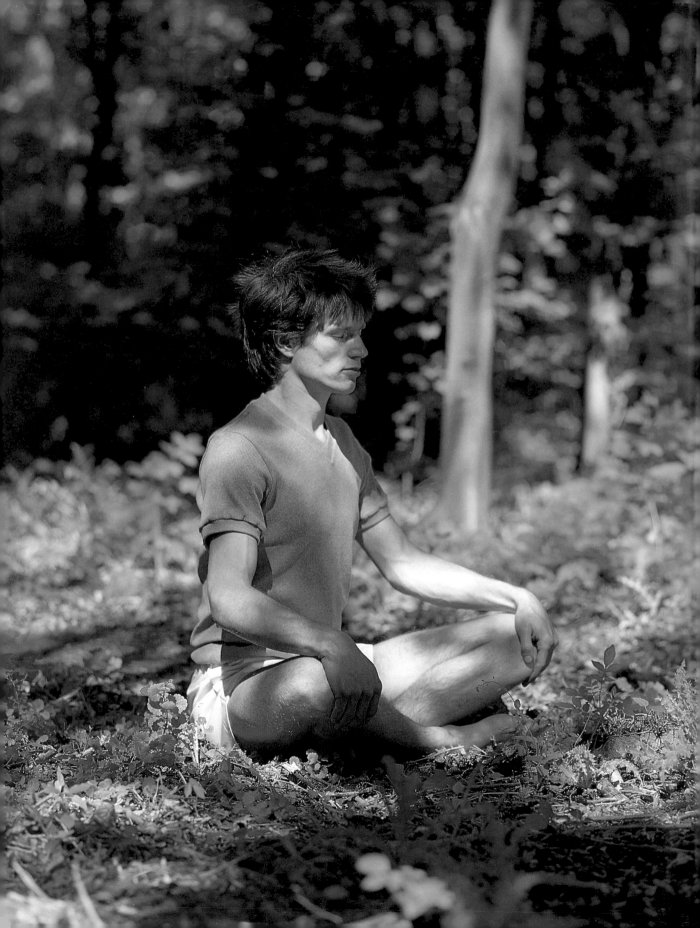

STEP-BY-STEP
YOGA
FOR STRESS RELIEF

SWAMI SHIVAPREMANANDA

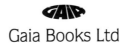

Gaia Books Ltd

A GAIA ORIGINAL

Books from Gaia celebrate the vision of Gaia, the self-sustaining living Earth, and seek to help its readers live in greater personal and planetary harmony.

Designer	Phil Gamble
Editor	Clare Stewart
Editorial Supervisor	Jo Godfrey Wood
Illustration	Peter Mennim, Mark Preston
Photography	Andrew Rumball
Managing Editor	Pip Morgan
Production	Lyn Kirby
Direction	Patrick Nugent
Consultant	Jane Sill
Contributor	Ruth Gilmore, Yoga Biomedical Trust

®This is a Registered Trade Mark of Gaia Books
an imprint of Octopus Publishing Group
2-4 Heron Quays, London E14 4JP

This edition published in 2000
First published in the United Kingdom in 1998 by
Gaia Books Ltd.

ISBN 1 85675 126 0

A catalogue record of this book is available from the British Library.

Printed and bound in China

10 9 8 7 6 5 4 3

Caution

Yoga can be practised by people of all ages and states of fitness.

Always observe the cautions given, and consult a doctor if you are in doubt about a medical condition.

When practising the postures and breathing exercises, work through each step gradually, and never rush any movement. Always be aware of your physical limits, and if you are a beginner only do as much as feels comfortable. Never try to force yourself into any position.

If you do hurt yourself, massage the area and stop the posture for a day. Resume when you feel ready.

There are a few postures and breathing exercises to be avoided if you have a specific medical condition, or which you should only do under the guidance of a yoga therapist. These are all clearly indicated throughout the text.

CONTENTS

HOW TO USE THIS BOOK

The book is made up of three parts. Part One has two chapters: the first deals with the psychology of stress while the second looks at the physiology of stress. Part Two, which forms the body of the book, consists of the Three-Month Programme – a practical programme of yoga exercises, breathing techniques and meditation exercises for you to follow. Part Three deals with specific ailments, and gives advice on which postures and breathing exercises to practise from the Three-Month Programme to alleviate your particular condition.

Chapter One explains how we can learn to manage stress by changing our attitudes and ways of behaviour. This section discusses the formative influences which shape us as children and which are partly responsible for creating our personalities as adults. The author offers suggestions on how to deal with past experiences which may have been damaging, and how to develop a positive attitude to life. He also looks at other causes for stress, such as environmental factors and emotional factors.

The fundamental message of Chapter One is that you have to gain an understanding of yourself in order to manage stress. You should try to carry this understanding with you throughout your practise of the Three-Month Programme.

Chapter Two explains how stress affects the body in physical terms. This part deals with the physiological changes which occur when the mind and body are under stress – how stress affects the nervous system, the organs of the body and the immune system. The author indicates how to recognise the various warning signals which show you are stressed, and suggests ways to manage your stress or alleviate stress-related disorders.

CAUTION
Throughout the Three-Month Programme wherever there is any need to avoid practising a particular posture or breathing exercise, a caution will appear in a highlighted circle.

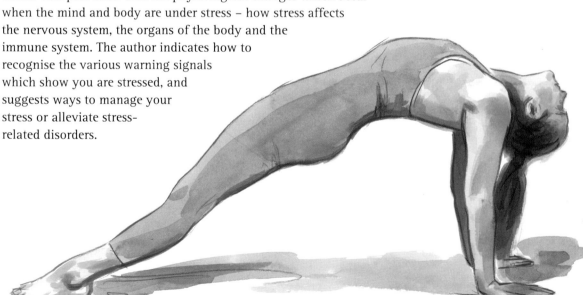

Part Two, the Three-Month Programme, is divided into six fortnightly parts. The Programme has step-by-step, fully illustrated instructions on how to perform the postures, breathing exercises and meditations. It opens with some easy postures and gradually introduces more demanding exercises. People of all ages and states of fitness can use the Programme, and it can be adapted to your own individual needs.

Part Three focuses on certain stress-related ailments and conditions, indicating which *asanas* and *pranayamas* are appropriate to relieve stress. The ailments covered include such commonplace conditions as insomnia, headaches, asthma, depression and hypertension. To assist you with using this section there is a reference chart (see p.121) which indicates which postures, breathing exercises and meditation practices you should focus on, or avoid, for each ailment.

At the back of the book you will find a list of useful texts for further reading and a resources section which gives information on yoga courses and centres where you can study several branches of yoga and train to become a teacher. These include courses on *Hatha* yoga, Remedial yoga, Iyengar yoga and yoga of the Sivananda School. The glossary includes all the Sanskrit terms used throughout the book and any other words that may require further clarification.

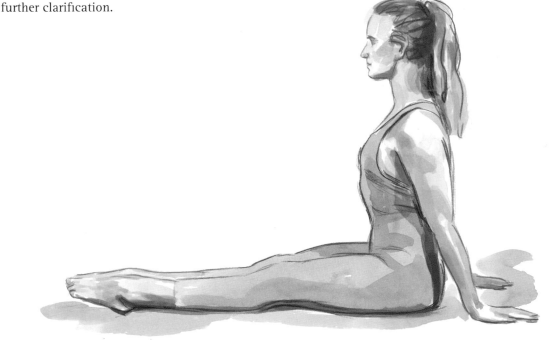

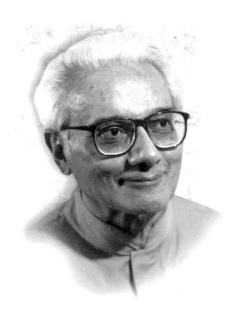

INTRODUCTION

Although born a *brahmin*, my upbringing was secular and I had a Western education. My parents instilled in me that ambition was a legitimate goal and that it was essential to develop the intellect in order to succeed. As a result, I entered university at the precocious age of fifteen. At the time I was totally unaware of the existence of stress. However, academic pressure made me an introvert. To escape from these pressures I dreamt of the explorers' tales of strange lands such as the Amazon and Tibet, of failed expeditions to Mount Everest (in the late 1930s), and of the mysterious knight-errants of the spirit in the high Himalayas.

Even at that age I was planning to explore the Himalayas, blissfully oblivious of the resources needed. I was hoping to discover whether there really existed sages from whose direct wisdom I could gain an insight into the mystery of life, and yogis whose ability to attain mastery over mind would help me to discipline my restless spirit. My studies, however, were intended to prepare me for a career in the civil service or foreign office. I was rational enough to know that I was merely a callous adolescent and my flights of imagination did not amount to much. I had no plans or qualifications for entering into a monastic life. I was not interested in the physical aspect of *Hatha* yoga. My fascination lay in the search for the inner spirit.

In the bustling cities of India, the poor struggled to eke out a living, including the lower-middle classes – the strain manifest on their faces. The small upper-middle class and the rich imitated the West, with little concern for the poor, and did not look very happy either. Nearly fifty-five years ago India was not as suffocatingly overpopulated as it is now. Eighty per cent of the population lived in villages, where life was serene and in harmony with nature. The physical hardship of the peasants, and the lack of modern amenities, did not appear to take its toll. They seemed to accept life philosophically and to maintain an inner calm, in contrast to what I had been taught – to be extremely ambitious. I decided instead that I could prove my worth by being useful to society, and yet refuse to be consumed by ambition.

At the age of nineteen, it was one of those inexplicable quirks of destiny that led me to Rishikesh, in the foothills of the Central Himalayas, where I met Swami Sivananda, and was invited to stay at his monastery. My intention was to spend a couple of weeks there and to return home, but I ended up staying more than sixteen years. Under this remarkable teacher I studied the major branches of yoga, and served as one of his personal secretaries throughout. It was here that I had the opportunity to meet the many visitors who came to learn about yoga, and who had come to stay for a while in a peaceful place. Many of these people had stress-related health problems. I observed that during their time in the *ashram* they developed an understanding of how to alleviate their stress. This was through looking at its causes, and using the practice of meditation, *asanas* (postures) and *pranayamas* (breathing exercises) to alleviate the symptoms.

In 1961 the Swami Sivananda sent me to the West to spread the teachings of yoga, firstly to the United States, and then to South America and Europe. Since then I have established several yoga centres in both the Americas, and teach several other smaller groups in Western Europe. For several years I taught *Hatha* yoga,

Raja yoga and the Vedanta philosophy to hundreds of students, both as the director of the Sivananda Yoga-Vedanta Centre of New York, and in the rest of the USA and in Canada.

In 1962 I was invited to South America to set up the Sivananda Yoga-Vedanta Centres in Buenos Aires, Argentina, and Montevideo, Uruguay, and then in 1965 to Santiago in Chile. During my years of teaching I have had the privilege to observe how yoga has helped my students to keep physically fit and to manage stress-related problems. It is this teaching experience gained over 36 years that has helped me to devise a simple and effective programme for the alleviation and prevention of stress.

Yoga is about achieving a balanced mind – neither being swayed by too much ambition, nor dragged down by failure. Yoga teaches you not to over-value achievement, to take in your stride set-backs and to reassess, and push ahead with life. The practice of yoga can help you to find peace in having achieved your best.

I hope that this book will be useful to those who are willing to apply the spiritual values I speak of to their lives, and to make the practice of the simple postures, breathing exercises and meditation techniques a part of their lives. The key to success is to keep an open mind, to practise regularly with commitment and to learn from life's experience.

Shivapremananda

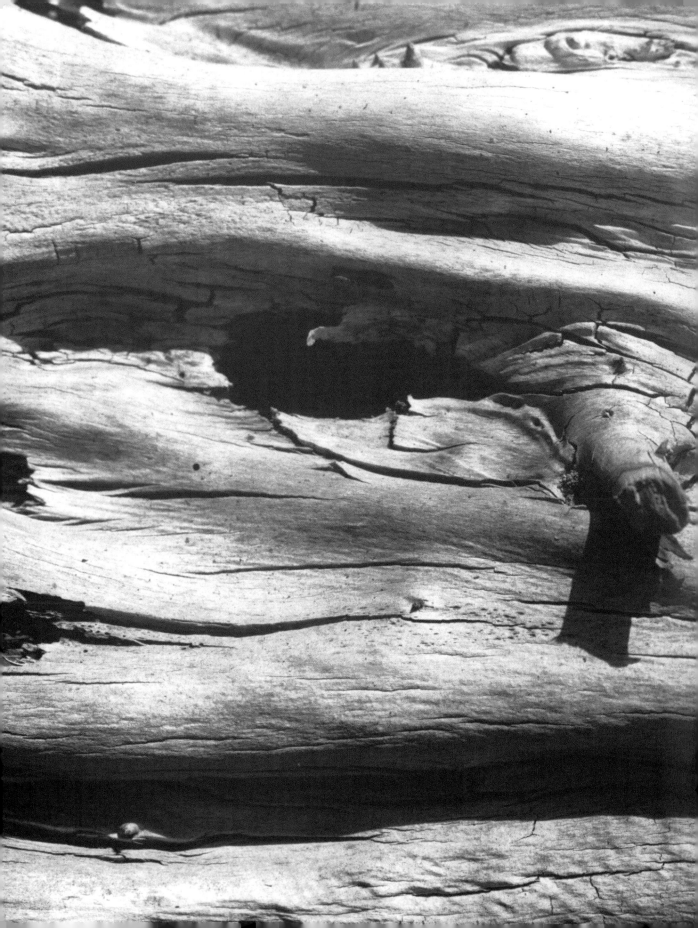

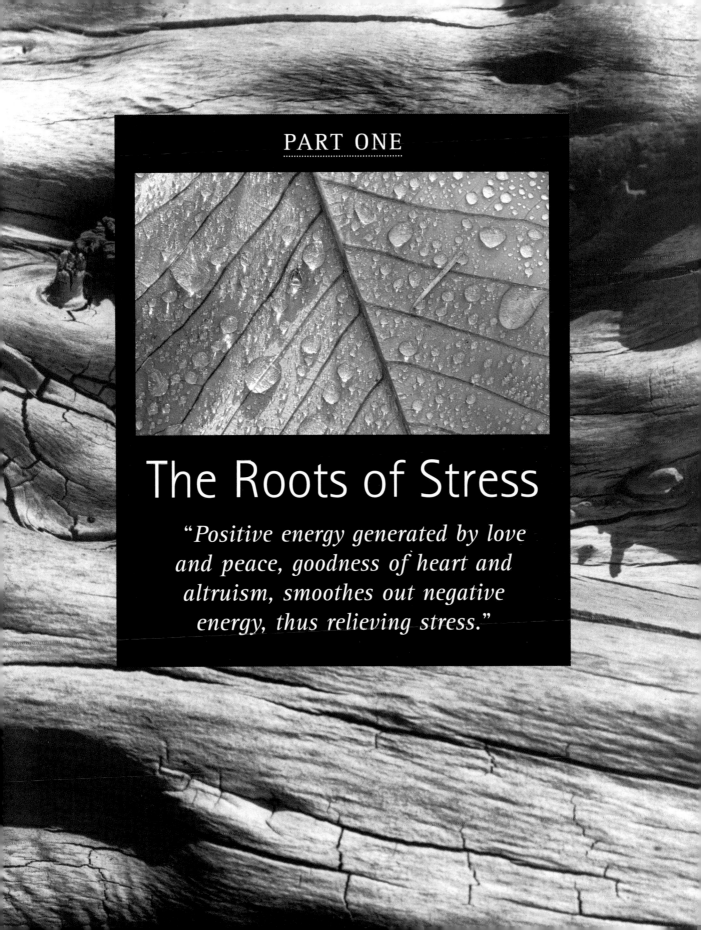

PART ONE

The Roots of Stress

"Positive energy generated by love and peace, goodness of heart and altruism, smoothes out negative energy, thus relieving stress."

CHAPTER ONE

The psychology of stress

Life consists of a series of involvements with others. We have parents, siblings and partners, and without involvement we cannot survive. While growing up we are dependent on others, and because of our lack of life experience we may respond to our circumstances in negative ways, which prevent us enjoying life and lead to a build up of stress.

In order to learn how to manage stress we have to understand its underlying causes. If we go to our doctor complaining of stress-related symptoms such as headaches and insomnia, he or she will probably treat the symptom on the surface, rather than looking at its deep-rooted psychological causes. However, he or she may take into account environmental factors.

To tackle stress you can practise yoga, and breathing and meditation exercises, but for long-term results you need to gain an understanding of the problems of human nature and learn how to cope with them.

In this first chapter of the book, I will deal with the psychological management of stress, while explaining its symptoms, causes and effects.

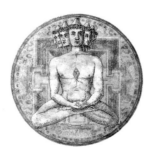

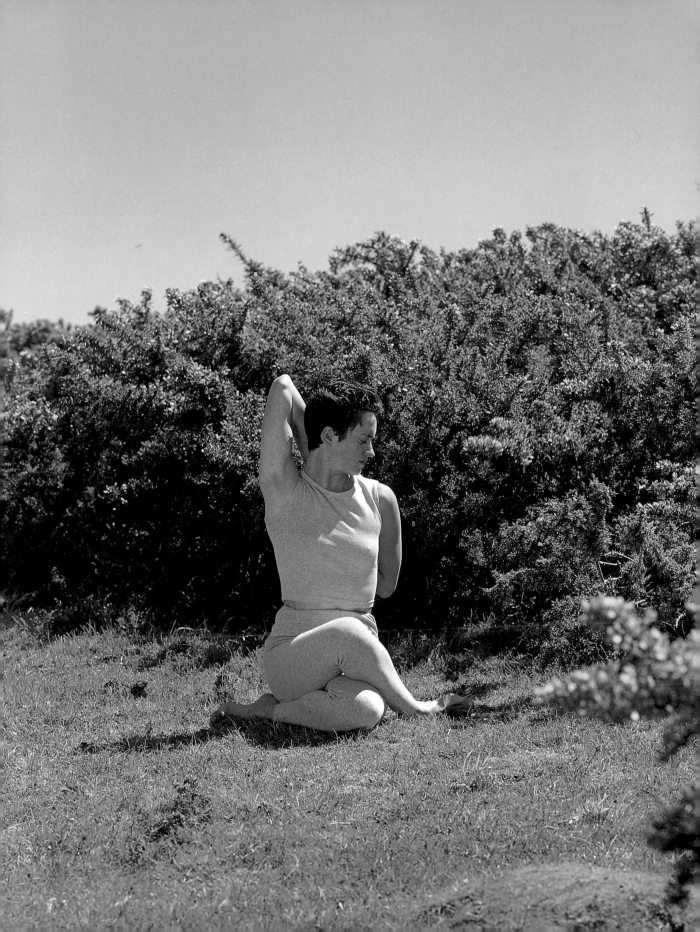

There are three main causes of stress: lack of love and security in childhood; environmental factors such as pollution and overcrowding in cities; and the triggering effect of a sudden event such as the death of a close relative or friend, failure in an examination, job loss or a financial debacle.

We all encounter stressful situations in our everyday lives. For example, we may need to meet deadlines at work, have to take an exam for which we are unprepared or have to face relationship difficulties. Similarly, a sudden cultural change, such as migrating to an unfamiliar country, or moving from a rural to a congested urban area, can cause stress.

In order to grow up emotionally healthy and be able to adapt to different situations in life, we need the nourishment of love, especially from our parents, because the first two years of a child's existence are most intimately related to them, and revolve around being really wanted and accepted, or not.

EARLY INSECURITIES

When a baby repeatedly cries for attention, it is already showing a sign of stress due to insecurity, wanting to be held in the arms of an adult, to feel protected through physical warmth and be looked at with a smile. Similarly, when a child regularly throws a tantrum, however unreasonably, on account of a frustrated whim, it is showing a sign of stress. A child who is persistently destructive, and cries continually, is expressing insecurity about parental love and apprehension that something has gone wrong between its parents. If we feel insecure about our parents' love for us as children, in later life we may find it difficult to develop a healthy relationship with a partner, and might suffer loneliness and even feelings of depression.

When trying to understand and treat stress-related physical and mental disorders, we often overlook how important it is to have had a secure background from the earliest stage in life. The emotional fulfilment we gain from being loved and understood is an antidote to stress. In order to create happy and loving relationships, we need to have a balanced sense of ourselves.

THE IMPORTANCE OF A SECURE UPBRINGING

A lack of role models in childhood is another factor which shapes our state of mind and is another basic cause of stress. Children need the presence of a parent or guardian with whom they can develop a one-to-one relationship, in order to grow into secure and happy individuals. Children who grow up without this may suffer stress in adult life. However, they can make up for this loss as adults, by finding resources within themselves to overcome stress.

If a child is brought up by adults who are dishonest, fail to keep promises, lack moral conviction and physical courage or are pretentious, careless and irresponsible, he will absorb these negative character traits. If he then demonstrates these characteristics in later life, and is humiliated by others for his weaknesses, he may feel very insecure and stressed.

PERSONALITY TYPES, SIGNS AND EFFECTS

Some of the environmental factors leading to stress include rapid urban development and industrialisation, leading to inner-city overcrowding. Those of us living in large cities are subject to the added pressures of having to hurry, and compete relentlessly. Changes in the employment-market have lead to increased job insecurity which is another cause for stress. Depending on their genetic make-up, some people are well equipped to cope with pressure while others find it more difficult to adapt.

There are two basic types of personality: extrovert and introvert. Psychologists define these as A and B types. Most of us have a combination of characteristics from both types. The A type is ambitious, enterprising, restless and hard-working. The B type is rather easy-going, less outwardly ambitious, prone to procrastination and sloth. The former is more likely to get stress-related ailments such as hypertension (see p.123), peptic ulcers (see p.124), cardiovascular disorders (see p.122), even diabetes (see p.125) – all the more so when genetically predisposed. The B type does not generally suffer from these physical effects but can be susceptible to psychological repercussions such as listlessness, death wish, insomnia and depression, due to lack of emotional fulfilment.

We can keep a look out for early stress signals such as nervousness, irritability, neck pain, shoulder and lower back pain, and disrupted sleep (see p.129). As our stress levels increase, our pulse rate and blood pressure go up. We may suffer loss of appetite or grow unnaturally hungry, sweat or feel cold. We may also experience an increase in stomach acidity, problems with digestion (see p.124), difficult bowel movements and sleeplessness (see p.129).

Allowing our stress to accumulate can cause outbursts of anger or violent behaviour. A persistent bad relationship in the family or at work will gradually lead us to experience corrosive frustration and gnawing anxiety, lack of will, indecisiveness and depression. Stress-related industrial and road accidents often occur after an explosive argument, or are caused by tension at work, fatigue or too much alcohol.

Heavy smokers are more likely to develop stress, despite the fact that many people say they smoke in order to relax. Addiction to alcohol and other stimulants can produce stressful reactions (see p.132). Suffering from persistent mental anguish that puts a strain on the nervous system (see p.130), can lead to hypertension (see p.123) and peptic ulcers (see p.124).

Living in an overcrowded home, having family difficulties, or being based in a noisy and congested neighbourhood with a lack of open and green space, will increase our sensitivity to stress and make us more irritable.

We can cause ourselves unnecessary stress if we are in a job which stretches us beyond our limits, or if we are over-ambitious, without having the necessary skills and drive to fulfil our ambition. In a similar way, persistent pressure to excel in our job, or criticism for not being successful enough, will cause us stress.

DEVELOPING A POSITIVE APPROACH TO LIFE

We all react to environmental factors differently, depending on our personality type, but our cultural background also plays a vital role. Spiritual faith can help us to accept what cannot be avoided. We will find it much easier to manage our stress if we are able to use adverse conditions in a positive way, to teach us how to improve our situation, and if we can practise detachment. This means distancing ourselves from a situation, so that we don't expend unnecessary energy on events beyond our control. By achieving these aims we will be less sensitive to environmental influences and therefore less susceptible to stress.

Emotional factors play a role in developing psychosomatic disorders. If we are feeling angry, resentful, afraid or sad, these emotions may cause stress-related symptoms. People who are easily irritated are more likely to develop cardiovascular (see p.122), digestive (see p.124) and respiratory ailments (see p.126). When we are angry or stressed we may restrict the flow of blood to the heart muscles, which can cause *angina pectoris*. Similarly, if we suffer from tension in the abdomen, the blood supply to the stomach is restricted, and can lead to excess gastric acid and peptic ulcers.

We can gain much relief from stress by unburdening our problems to a close friend or relative, but to be in proper control of our stress we have to understand our basic human nature and its psychological roots.

MANAGING THE INNER CAUSES OF STRESS

Stress results from selfishness and self-importance; the two sides of the primitive ego, the id. Egoism, concern for one's own interests and welfare, above all else, is really systematic selfishness, and selfishness can have long-lasting consequences. It can make us feel isolated and unloved, because it is hard for others to like and relate to a very selfish person. We are all selfish by nature, to a certain extent, and are therefore reluctant to take on board another person's selfish demands. Their self-centredness is an uncomfortable reminder of our own.

However, some people are less selfish than others. Some of us have the advantage of having being brought up to be considerate and responsible to others, because our parents have been good role models. Others of us lack this head start in life and have to struggle not to be selfish and irresponsible. If we are selfish by nature and have not been taught how to manage our ego, we are more likely to be irresponsible and unreliable, and we will fail to win people's trust. If others cannot trust us, we will cause ourselves added stress.

Selfishness is the natural expression of our instinct for survival. However, too much self-interest can make our lives empty by alienating us from others. We can become less selfish by learning to be considerate and useful to others. A selfish person tends to be over-sensitive to criticism and is easily offended, which makes him more susceptible to stress. By practising tolerance and detachment, we will make more space in our lives for others. These are the first steps towards managing the ego.

"Self-importance", believing that things revolve around us, is a form of self-defence, which can cause us stress. If we lack belief in what we are saying, we may try to compensate by insisting that we are always right and when others see through us, we will feel humiliated and full of stress.

To gain the respect and trust of others we must learn to manage our selfishness and "self-importance". By being honest and not taking ourselves too seriously, we can avoid unnecessary worry and stress, both to ourselves and others.

Feelings of hurt, self-pity and resentment can cause us stress. Resentment stems from self-pity, a tendency to avoid responsibility, and to blame others when things go wrong.

We have three deep-rooted needs in our psyche: the need to love and be loved by a few people with whom we can identify; the need to be fulfilled by work or activities we find enjoyable and rewarding; and the need to strive towards achieving our goals.

Developing healthy and balanced friendships and relationships helps us to feel emotionally fulfilled, and gives us a sense of purpose. Sharing our happiness with others, doing useful work, and trying to be a better person, can greatly lessen our stress. By sharing our lives with others we will be more fulfilled and happier people. If we have inner contentment, and a genuine love for life, we will be better equipped to manage our stress.

SELF-CENTREDNESS, VANITY AND PRIDE

To find happiness, we have to understand the selfish part of ourselves. The ego is what motivates us to survive and, through ambition and competition, enables us to progress and achieve our goals in life.

We can control our selfish instincts by making an effort to be generous rather than mean-spirited. By being open to new ideas and influences, and always ready to learn from our experiences, we can become less conceited. We need to develop the ability to see ourselves objectively. Feeling continually sorry for ourselves can lead to feelings of depression. We can avoid this by taking responsibility for ourselves, a liberating experience which will make our lives richer.

Self-centredness is another form of the ego that is different from selfishness. A self-centred person can be generous to those he or she cares for, but likes to be the centre of attention, and to receive appreciation and flattery. When he is not, he feels disappointed and frustrated and this causes stress.

Vanity is another cause of stress. Trying to win attention and esteem, because we look good, or want others to praise our successes, will put others off. When they reject us, we experience unhappiness and stress. What really matters is personal integrity. If you try to behave graciously by cultivating decency, compassion, honesty and sympathy, you will have no inclination to worry about your image.

Those of us who enjoy good friendships and happy relationships, and have the emotional support of others, can cope better with everyday pressures. When we are faced with a sudden crisis, such as unemployment, bereavement, the break up of a relationship, or a serious illness, if we are happily married, or have caring and understanding partners, we are less likely to need professional help, such as counselling or psychotherapy.

Pride is yet another form of self-importance. We are perfectly justified in taking pride in a friend or partner's success, but being excessively proud about our own achievements is a sign of superficiality. It suggests we are trying to hide an inferiority complex beneath conceit. It is a truism that those who are conscious of their virtue are not really virtuous. Those confident of their worth do not need to boast about their worthiness.

An undisciplined and unrefined ego is the root cause of psychological stress. Having a healthy and well-balanced ego helps us to make positive choices, and to achieve our goals. If we repress it, we are in danger of becoming indifferent and irresponsible. If we lack a proper sense of ourselves, we are more likely to be exploited by people with stronger and more cunning egos.

To find relief from stress, you have to understand the ego and master its many facets.

ATTACHMENT AND POSSESSIVENESS

Being totally dependent upon someone else, emotionally, can cause us intense anguish and stress. When we are passionately in love, the stronger our attachment is to the other person, the worse our pain will be when the relationship ends. Being unable to accept the fact that it is over, once and for all, prolongs our distress. Being excessively attached to someone else is a form of self-love. We want to possess the other person, and fail to realise that in doing so, we are loving ourselves.

Moving away from our normal environment, going on a long journey for example, or getting involved in some kind of interesting work, can help. We have to detach ourselves from the situation, to allow the wound to heal, and avoid wallowing in self-pity. The best solution is to throw ourself into something which will absorb our attention, such as an interest, or a creative activity, requiring a lot of mental energy.

We can try to practise detachment in our approach to life, as a means of preventing stress. This means letting go of our ego, so we can see things more clearly; putting things into perspective and being realistic about our situation. For example, if we stand too close to a mirror, we cannot see ourselves properly. Only by distancing ourselves can we gain a true perspective. Similarly when we are immersed in a problem, we lack the objectivity to solve it, and this can cause stress. Conversely, if we stand too far away from a mirror, we lose sight of ourselves. This is equivalent to indifference, avoiding responsibility, as opposed to detachment.

When we hold an object too tightly, we are aware of only the strength of our grip and are unable to feel its texture and weight.

This is the case with possessiveness in a relationship. We are conscious of only our ego, possessing the other person, and not of the person we seek to relate to, know and love.

JUDGING PEOPLE'S CHARACTERS

Another cause of stress is having unreasonable expectations of others. We are so fixated on ourselves that we fail to see what other people are really like and so develop false expectations of them. For example, we may hope that a very selfish person will be capable of love, or that someone who is generally unreliable will be capable of being responsible.

To keep our peace of mind and avoid disappointment, we have to be realistic about other people's potential, and observant about their character. When we take on a commitment involving someone else, to avoid disappointment, we need to make clear from the outset what each of our roles are. We also become stressed by going against the tide, such as refusing to adapt to another culture and way of life when we travel abroad.

Learning to manage our desires, approximating them to our needs, and matching our ambitions with our talents, are fundamental to our peace of mind. Desires arise from our need to live as enjoyably and successfully as possible. However, we need to take into consideration how well we are equipped to achieve what we desire.

THE AMBITIOUS PERSONALITY

People who are very ambitious need to have leadership qualities, and the kind of intelligence that allows them to focus on the job in hand, in order to fulfil their goals. They also need to be driven by a desire for serious hard work and commitment. Highly ambitious people are more likely to suffer from physical stress. This is because they have a tendency to push themselves beyond their limits, without giving themselves sufficient rest. This drive to succeed takes its toll on their bodies.

Very high achievers may be more susceptible to illnesses such as strokes and heart disease (see p.122). Whereas those who have unrealistic goals, and lack the necessary qualities to achieve them, could be prone to psychological stress, such as anxiety and lack of self-esteem, for failing to achieve.

We have to accept that only one person in ten is a born leader, and that the rest of us have to settle with taking second place – a position which is just as valuable and rewarding.

KEEPING OUR MINDS ACTIVE

There are two types of success, material and spiritual, and we should strive for both. We work hard so we can have the security, say, of having our own home. Apart from wanting material comfort, we also need spiritual security. Our homes are places where we can enjoy the warmth and love of a family or a close relationship, and a sense of belonging among those we live with.

One of the most effective means of countering stress is to avoid boredom. We need to find ways of keeping our minds active. The more stressed we are, the faster we will age physically, whereas the normal ageing process accelerates from the time we lose interest in life. To keep our minds healthy, we should have something to look forward to - an interesting place to visit, a different culture to get acquainted with, a new area of knowledge to explore, some latent talent to develop.

Above all, we should have some spiritual goals to realise, such as striving to be a more caring, supportive, loyal and loving friend or companion, with more patience and tolerance, and trying to gain a greater understanding of the foibles of human nature, while correcting them in ourselves.

OVERCOMING STRESS

By using the self-help methods I have suggested, you can learn to deal with your stress. Acquiring self-discipline, and developing a new philosophical outlook on life, will help you to overcome stress. If you try to understand the complexities of human nature, and learn to deal with them, you will be more than half-way to overcoming your stress.

By far the hardest part of managing your stress is learning a new psychological approach to your life. This is the real challenge. However, a much easier way of coping with stress is through physical exercise, such as the simple stretches and postures, breathing exercises and calming meditations, which follow in Part Two.

These exercises can be done by anyone, of any age, in gradual stages. From the Three-Month Programme (see pp.35-117), select a suitable combination of exercises to suit your needs, depending on your physical fitness. By practising them, you will not only lessen your stress but prevent its occurring in the first place, and will generally keep healthy.

Take time to consider your thoughts. Overcome negative thinking.
When you find yourself thinking about someone negatively, try to
bring to mind something positive about them.

Be more conscious of your behaviour. If you are lying, try to correct
yourself. Personal integrity is more important than gaining a dubious
advantage over someone.

When you feel angry, try to be patient, and not to lose your temper.

Expect more from yourself than from others.

Think about the good qualities of someone you love, not on
your terms but on theirs; then try to help them.

Avoid self-justification. If you are right, there is no need to justify
yourself, whereas if you are wrong, you cannot afford to do so.

Learn to be adaptable, to adjust to different situations and
accommodate others, without losing your bearings.

Avoid deceit and hypocrisy by saying what you mean and
not exaggerating or belittling others.

Learn from your experience.

When evaluating your situation consider the facts, rather
than indulging in wishful thinking. The first requirement
for truth is evidence.

When making choices, take long-term consequences into
consideration, not short-term results.

Avoid secrecy as this can lead to deception.

Avoid prejudice and infatuation through practising fairness
and objectivity, and by being honest about the person.

Avoid impulsive behaviour. You won't make misjudgements and mistakes.

Try not to dwell in the past and spend time regretting lost friendships.
Instead help others with understanding, sympathy and friendship.
Accept the reality gracefully and do not lose your dignity.

Keep healthy through exercise, which will improve your breathing,
and therefore help you to think more clearly and creatively.

Look for a job which you will genuinely enjoy and commit
yourself to it. Find something creative to do, to keep your mind
occupied, and to build up your confidence and sense of purpose.

Learning to cope with the psychological causes of stress is not easy. It is not
always possible to control your circumstances or to manage others' feelings
towards yourself. However you can try to behave reasonably and not overreact.

CHAPTER TWO

The physiology of stress

Holistic approaches to health fully acknowledge the integration of the mind and body. The wellbeing of one depends on the good health of the other. At the same time, whatever disturbs the balance of one upsets the equilibrium of the other. Stress affects our whole being, yet we cannot live without it – it is part of being human. But the art is keeping stress manageable and positive. As soon as it becomes out of control – because it is persistent or extreme – we start to feel its negative effects.

Yoga can help us to control our stress and keep it at a manageable and useful level. It provides a trustworthy platform for relieving our minds and bodies from the adverse effects of stress. Chapter One has made clear the psychological roots of stress and indicates the kind of stress-related ailments that may result. The practice of yoga has the unique ability of preventing psychological stress from building up; it can also help to restore equilibrium to the physiological systems that stress upsets. In order to provide an understanding of this physiology, Chapter Two highlights the roles played by our nerves and hormones in our bodies' self-regulating approach to coping with stress. This chapter lays the groundwork for understanding how stress affects the body's systems, particularly the respiratory, digestive, endocrine and cardiovascular systems.

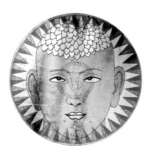

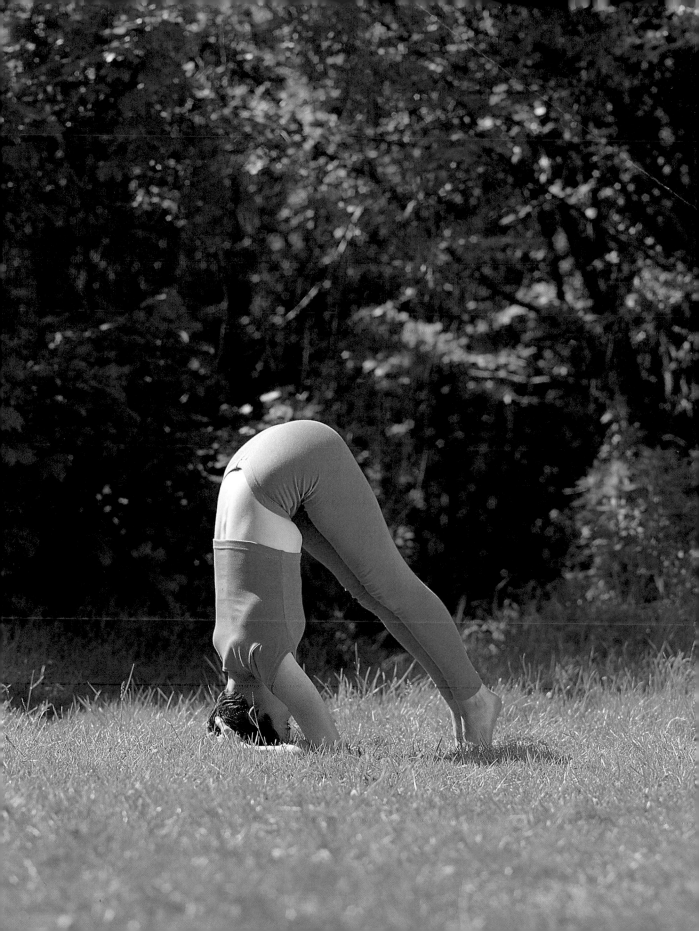

A STABLE MICROENVIRONMENT

All the body systems co-operate together throughout life to maintain inside the body a stable microenvironment, in which all the multiplicity of cells can survive and function to optimum effect. This microenvironment is usually very different from the outside world in terms of variables such as temperature, acidity and water concentration, and this difference is maintained by the constant adjustment of the variables within narrow limits.

The body will respond in a generalised non-specific way to any factor which overwhelms, or threatens to overwhelm, this maintained environment. The causes of the stress (the stressors) can affect the body at a physical or psychological level. Physical stressors include injury, severe exercise, and marked extremes of temperature, and sleep deprivation, while psychological and emotional states such as anxiety, grief and fear will also induce the stress response.

The primary stress or stimulus need not necessarily be unpleasant – events or factors which are regarded generally as being enjoyable may also involve underlying stressful elements, such as anxiety, decision-making or geographic relocation. For example, getting married has been ranked as being almost as stressful as redundancy from work, and moving house as almost as stressful as having problems with the boss.

The nature of the stress is not as important as the amount of it. It is natural for people to experience some stress in life, indeed stress often has the effect of producing an increase in the level of performance. It is only when the amount of stress exceeds an individual's tolerance level that performance starts to decline. People vary enormously in the amount of stress that they can cope with, and for any individual, the tolerance level can vary markedly at different stages of life.

THE STRESS RESPONSE

It is helpful to summarise the generalised stress response as the "fright, fight or flight" reaction. This description encapsulates the main response options open to an individual when interacting with, in particular, physical stress, and also suggests some of the physiological mechanisms which will be dominant in the chosen response. Some degree of apprehension or fear ("fright") is the usual subjective experience of the stress response. It is often necessary to decide whether to confront the stressor ("fight"), or whether to take avoiding action ("flight"), both the latter responses requiring the rapid activation of skeletal muscle, together with a high degree of increased performance in both the cardiovascular and the respiratory systems.

The stress response is entirely appropriate in an acute situation, where an increased level of performance can result. A stage performance, competitive sport or any type of emergency – all warrant such a stress response, and this is considered entirely normal. During or soon after the event, the response rapidly diminishes, and the physiological mechanisms effecting "fright, fight or flight" decline to normal values.

However, in modern everyday life most of the common stressors that we experience are not predominantly physical, but are more psychosocial in nature, such as work stress, job insecurity and worry about family problems. The generalised stress response is not so appropriate here, and the often chronic nature of the stressor or stressors can lead to a permanent state of heightened physical and psychological tension.

RECOGNISING THE STRESS SIGNS

Very often the onset of such chronic stress is quite insidious. With time, the individual adapts to the gradually changing state of the body and mind, unaware of the increasing burden of physical and mental tension. Yoga is of tremendous value as a therapy in this situation, as regular yoga practice leads to a heightened awareness of the self, which will enable the individual to discriminate more clearly between tension and relaxation. Recognition of the difference between these two states is the first step towards becoming empowered to effect changes in the lifestyle in order to reduce exposure to stressors, and the body's over-sensitive responses to them.

Signs of increasing stress can be physical or mental in type. Nervous mannerisms, such as biting the nails, repetitively clicking a pen or tapping the foot betray an inner state of unease, while a number of medical conditions, such as asthma and hypertension often are associated with the long-term stress response. These stress-related illnesses may be either caused by chronic stress, or worsened by it.

Although no scientifically acceptable cause-and-effect relationship has yet been proved in most cases, there is strong circumstantial evidence linking chronic exposure to stress with such conditions as repetitive strain injury, irritable bowel syndrome and some types of low back pain. Behavioural and psychological disorders associated with chronic stress range from mild anxiety or depression to the complete collapse of all coping mechanisms usually referred to as a nervous breakdown.

Individuals suffering from stress-related diseases sometimes find it difficult to find effective medical help, as the time required for a family doctor or consultant to provide the long-term counselling type of support needed in such cases often is not readily available.

Over-stressed people use a variety of coping mechanisms in order to try to ease their plight. The occasional cigarette, alcoholic drink or sleeping tablet can be the start of a downward spiral into addiction and/or substance abuse, which then has to be coped with in addition to the original stressors. Eating disorders, such as anorexia and bulimia, also can develop as albeit unsuccessful attempts to manage an otherwise unbearable situation.

NERVES AND HORMONES

Stress affects many components of the neuroendocrine system of nerves and hormones, and as a result, secondary changes take place in the activity and function of most of the body's organs. For example, heart rate increases dramatically and the liver releases some of its store of energy-rich glycogen. Before considering these changes in more detail, it is necessary to examine some of the component parts of this integrated system.

The nervous system consists of a complex arrangement of nerve cells (neurones), which transmit information to one another by the release and uptake from cell to cell of small messenger molecules called neurotransmitters. These chemicals carry messages over the small distances between adjacent neurones, thus activating in turn the individual members of the inter-connecting chains of nerve cells forming the numerous pathways in the nervous system.

The endocrine system consists of cells and organs which release small messenger molecules (hormones) into the blood stream, in order to affect the functioning of other cells or tissues some distance away.

In the past, the nervous and endocrine systems were considered to be separate entities, although it has been long accepted that they interacted. There are important similarities between the two systems: first, they are both concerned with communication and integration in the body; second, they both rely on the use of numerous small messenger molecules; and third, their functioning is interdependent at many levels throughout the body.

These three similarities have led to the acceptance of a new, more holistic concept within physiology – that of the neuroendocrine system, a single communications network that is responsible for much of the integrated working of the body.

OUR SELF-GOVERNING NERVOUS SYSTEM

The autonomic nervous system supplies motor and sensory innervation to involuntary muscle (such as is found in the walls of many blood vessels, in the gut, in the respiratory tract and in the heart), and to most of the glands of the body. "Autonomic" means "self-governing", and indicates that the nerve cells belonging to this system are responsible for the subconscious regulation and execution of many of the routine day-to-day activities which maintain the constant internal environment. The autonomic nervous system is of primary importance in the individual's responses to stress, so it is necessary to consider its layout and function in more detail.

The autonomic nervous system has two component parts, which work together in the execution of some physiological processes, but which also can act in a more independent way when required. The two parts of the system are called sympathetic and parasympathetic.

Sympathetic activity forms an important part of the stress response, and this also has secondary effects on the parasympathetic side, which is primarily responsible for the maintenance of much of the routine, day-to-day involuntary activity of the body. As in the rest of the nervous system, autonomic motor activity is initiated and controlled by the brain. The part of the brain around the hypothalamus (the limbic area) is particularly associated with the emotions and has widespread effects in association with both the autonomic nervous system and the nearby pituitary gland.

The parasympathetic motor distribution is confined to the head and the organs within the trunk, while sympathetic nerve fibres supply the limbs as well as the rest of the body. Because of this, activation of the sympathetic system results in a widespread stress reaction which also is inseparably intertwined with concomitant activation of the hormone-producing endocrine organs, such as the pituitary, adrenals, thyroid and reproductive glands.

THE ENDOCRINE SYSTEM

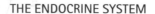

...ne body is particularly vulnerable to
...ef introduction to how stress affects the
...ne seven main endocrine glands follows.

pituitary gland

...a small region of the brain that acts as a major
...l of body temperature and appetite. Its complex
...ith the cerebral cortex, and with other parts of
...e little understood, link emotions with the body's
...is system.

...land, a pea-sized structure rather like an upside-
down ... n, hangs by a stalk from the undersurface of the
brain. By producing a range of controller hormones it orchestrates
the secretion of hormones from the other endocrine glands of the
body – for example, cortisol from the adrenal glands. Because the
hypothalamus controls the activity of the pituitary gland, it
indirectly masterminds this orchestration.

Stress increases the activity of the hypothalamus which, in its
turn, instructs the pituitary gland to increase the secretion of
hormones responsible for the stress response. The pituitary releases
controlling hormones, particularly the adrenocorticotrophic
hormone (ACTH) – see the adrenal glands, below.

The adrenal glands

The adrenal glands perch, like little hats, one on the top of each
kidney. Each gland has two parts, an outer cortex and an inner
medulla. Partly in response to the ACTH from the pituitary (see
above) the cortex secretes a number of steroid hormones that
directly affect the balance of salt, water and glucose in the body.

The primary cortical hormone affecting glucose metabolism is
called cortisol. Cortisol is normally secreted by the adrenal cortex
according to a daily sleep/wake cycle. Its concentration in the
blood is at a much higher level during the day than at night.

During the stress response, cortisol secretion rises in proportion
to the degree of stress – this is most marked when the stress results
from a serious physical injury. By breaking down protein and fats
as well as carbohydrates, cortisol produces an increase in the
concentration of glucose in the blood. Stress, therefore, raises blood
sugar. This is an appropriate response to acute stress for it ensures
an adequate energy supply, for both brain and skeletal muscles, at a
time when immediate physical activity may be required.

As well as ACTH, the pituitary produces endorphins and other related compounds. The precise mode of operation of these substances is not yet clear. It may be that their pain-relieving properties, along with other postulated effects on mood and perception, may combine to allow life-saving exertion despite serious injury, as in many acts of heroism.

The adrenal medulla is intimately associated with the sympathetic nervous system. Its main secretion – adrenaline – is related to noradrenaline, one of the most important neurotransmitters of the sympathetic system. Adrenaline secretion is initiated by direct stimulation of the adrenal medulla by the sympathetic nerves.

Exposure to a stressor produces an immediate increase in sympathetic nerve activity, which in turn results in the release into the blood stream of significant quantities of adrenaline from the adrenal medulla. This hormone, being in the blood, can quickly permeate the tissues of the body, augmenting the activity of sympathetic nerves.

The effects are well known – raised heart rate and breathing rate, pallor, trembling, the hair standing on end. Along with these predominantly physical responses, feedback to the brain arouses the emotional response to stress, normally some degree of fearfulness and anxiety.

The thyroid gland

The thyroid gland is shaped like a butterfly or a bow tie, and sits across the front of the upper part of the trachea (windpipe). The cells of the thyroid manufacture hormones which are released into the blood stream in order to control the rate of metabolism in all the other tissues and organs (metabolism is the term used to describe the process of oxygen uptake and subsequent production of energy and heat within the body).

The thyroid normally stores within itself around three months supply of the hormones. This is a unique feature, as other endocrine glands usually only manufacture their secretory products as and when required. In most people thryoid hormone output is controlled within fairly narrow limits, but severe stressor exposure may result in increased production.

The pancreas

Much of the pancreas is non-endocrine in nature, being concerned with producing digestive juices for the gut. It is situated behind the stomach, and embedded within the bulk of the tissue lie numerous clusters of endocrine cells, the islets, which secrete insulin and glucagon, two substances with essentially complementary actions in the maintenance of normal blood glucose levels. Insulin lowers the blood sugar by encouraging the body's cells to absorb more glucose. Glucagon, on the other hand, raises blood sugar levels by mobilising the sizeable store of carbohydrate present in the liver and converting it to glucose.

Stress has important and marked effects on blood sugar regulation. Apart from the effects of increased cortisol secretion described above, adrenaline inhibits insulin secretion, thus allowing blood glucose levels to rise. This response is appropriate as part of the generalised "fright, fight or flight" reaction, as it will ensure that adequate levels of energy will be made available to carry out an appropriate response to the stressor.

The testes and ovaries

The testes and ovaries play a very important role as hormone-secreting endocrine organs in addition to the production of sperm and egg cells. In both sexes the manufacture and release of sex hormones during reproductive life is controlled by the hypothalamus and pituitary, in much the same way as they control the other endocrine organs.

It is well accepted that both acute and chronic stress can affect the hormonal balance of the female reproductive system. Irregularities of the menstrual cycle and disturbance or inhibition of ovulation occur commonly in the presence of both physical and emotional stressors. These effects usually are the result of imbalances at hypothalamic or pituitary level, since increased levels of cortisol secretion have an inhibitory effect on the brain.

Men are affected also by stress, with psycho-social factors being commonly responsible for episodes of sexual dysfunction, such as difficulties with erection or premature ejaculation. Although research findings are somewhat inconclusive, it seems reasonable to consider that sperm production might be affected by chronic stress.

The pineal gland

This small organ lies deep within the brain. It contains a hormone called melatonin, which is believed to be important in maintaining sleep/wake cycles and associated daily rhythms (such as cortisol secretion) in synchrony with the dark/light cycle. The balance of this delicate rhythm is easily upset by events such as

changing time zones, going on night duty and other causes of
sleep disturbance.

The thymus gland

The thymus is still referred to in some texts as a gland, but it is now
accepted that its primary role is as an important component of the
immune system. The thymus is most active before birth and during
early life, after which it becomes much smaller. Some researchers
believe that despite its size in adult life, its activity, especially its
continuing secretion of the hormone thymosin, remains significant.

The thymus is responsible for the initiation and maintenance of
an essential component of the immune response. It produces and
programmes a type of white blood cell (T cells), so that they can
distinguish between the body's own proteins and others of
"foreign" structure, such as those from invading bacteria or from
genetically-mutated cells. When the immune system identifies such
"foreign" proteins it can mobilise the resources to destroy and
remove them. Thymosin is involved in the maintenance of T cell
function. Maldevelopment or malfunction of this system may lead
to overwhelming infection, or the uncontrolled multiplication of
mutated cells, which may then become manifest as cancer.

Although it is commonly believed that exposure to chronic stress
reduces the immune response, the mechanisms through which such
an effect might operate are not clear. Stress does result in increased
levels of circulating adrenal steroids, such as cortisol, but those
produced by psychological stress are far below the concentration in
the blood needed to produce a measurable immunosuppressive
effect. Synthetic steroids similar to cortisol are used therapeutically
in order to suppress the immune response – for example to prevent
rejection after organ transplantation – but the doses are enormous
compared to those produced naturally by the body.

It is possible that the much lower levels of naturally occurring
steroids might exert a similar, smaller effect if maintained over a
long period of time, but this remains as yet unproven. It has been
found that while prolonged severe exercise suppresses normal
immune responses, moderate regular exercise enhances them.
Thus most forms of physical activity, which in excess can act as a
harmful stressor, will increase health and wellbeing when enjoyed
in moderation.

PART TWO

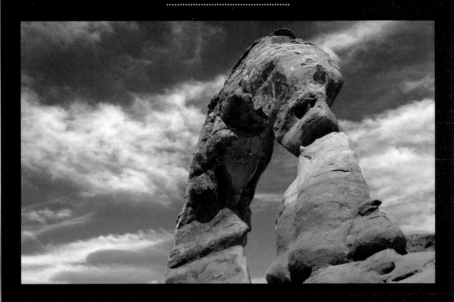

The Three-Month Programme

"The key to success is motivation, regular and committed practice, keeping an open mind and learning from experience."

THE THREE-MONTH PROGRAMME

The Three-Month Programme for stress relief is divided into six fortnightly parts. It opens with a series of stretches which loosen up your body and prepare you for the rest of the postures. These initial stretches, which you learn in the first two weeks, are repeated throughout each fortnight and form the basis of your practice.

The Programme is suitable for people of all ages and varied fitness. You will probably experience some discomfort when you first begin. This will depend largely on your state of fitness and your age. However, the basic postures at the outset are designed to allow your body to adapt to a schedule of exercise, and to ease any stiffness in the joints and tension in your limbs. As you progress through each fortnight the postures become gradually more demanding. However, with daily practice you will be surprised at how quickly you develop flexibility. People who are already flexible will be able from the outset to practise the classical postures in the later stages without difficulty.

The first fortnight consists of a basic half-hour session, which you can do even if you are very stiff. If at first your muscles ache, be patient with yourself. Keep in mind how many years it has taken for the tension to accumulate, and allow time for them to loosen up gradually. Follow the stretches involving the upper part of the body with a short relaxation in the lying-down position known as the Corpse Pose (*Shavasana*). You then continue with two simple breathing exercises which are especially good for stress alleviation. The concluding part of the session consists of a simple meditation, which will help to prepare your mind for your yoga practice.

The second fortnight opens with a series of additional stretches involving the lumbar region. If you have a stiff lower back and hamstring muscles you can begin by practising only half of the sequence and progress to completing it all once you are more flexible. The rest of the session is the same as in the first fortnight and will take a total of forty minutes.

In the third fortnight you learn one of the major classical *asanas*, the Shoulderstand and its related postures. You then practise a relaxation technique, and continue with two standard breathing exercises (*pranayamas*) for stress alleviation from the first fortnight. You end the session with two more *pranayamas*, *Shitali* and *Shitakari*, particularly effective at calming the mind, followed by a meditation which will help you achieve a deeper relaxation.

The fourth fortnight opens with the the Bowing-Down Pose and the Half-Headstand, followed by the Child Pose. These postures where your head is resting on the ground are very beneficial for stress relief. You then repeat the breathing exercises from the first fortnight, *Nadi-Sodhana* and *Ujjayi*, and conclude with a meditation. The session will take three-quarters of an hour.

The fifth fortnight focuses upon an all-round and more vigorous form of exercise, the twelve Salutations to the Sun. You combine this sequence with a more vigorous form of breathing exercise, *Kapalabhati*, which replaces the two previous *pranayamas*, *Shitali* and *Shitakari*. You finish with the meditation from weeks one and two, followed by a new meditative practice. In this last meditation you chose certain phrases to help affirm your belief in the practice.

In the last fortnight, you can increase your practice from two to four rounds of the Sun Salutation. You continue with the same breathing exercises as in the previous fortnight, but replace the meditation with a much deeper form of relaxation known as *Yoga Nidra*. The whole session will require about an hour and a quarter.

The whole of the Three-Month Programme is accompanied by step-by-step illustrations and clear instructions to guide you through each exercise. There are useful tips throughout the text which give you basic advice about yoga practice, and cautions to warn you which postures or breathing exercises to avoid if you have a certain condition. So even if you are a beginner you can proceed with confidence. Be aware of your body's limits and never push yourself beyond your capacity.

When first learning the postures it helps to concentrate on each step in turn. After a few months practice you will find yourself memorising the sequences. When practising do not be tempted to rush through the postures. It is important to breathe slowly and deeply in each stage of the posture. There are several breathing exercises throughout the Programme which teach you to do this. There are four stages to all major *asanas*. Preparing for the posture by loosening up your body, moving into the posture and holding it while breathing slowly and deeply, controlled movement in the posture in rhythm with your breath, and coming out of the pose.

By beginning with the simple exercises from the opening fortnight and slowly building up to the more vigorous and demanding exercises in the last fortnights, you will find yourself mastering the Programme without difficulty. With commonsense and perseverance and unfailing regular practice, you can use this comprehensive Three-Month Programme not only to help alleviate your stress but to prevent it as well.

PLANNING YOUR DAY'S PRACTICE
When planning your day's practice, you could start with the shoulder stretches and neck movements from weeks one and two (see pp.40-51) followed by the lumbar stretches from weeks three and four (see pp.60-9). Lie in *Shavasana* (see p.52) for three minutes and continue with two to four rounds of the Sun Salutation (see pp.108-9). Follow with the Shoulderstand (pp.72-7) and Cobra series (pp.94-105), relaxing in *Shavasana* for a few minutes between. Choose two or three *pranayamas* to conclude your practice. Rest in *Shavasana* for at least 10 minutes, covering yourself with a blanket.

CHAPTER THREE

Weeks one and two

There are three groups of exercises which you can use daily as the basis of your yoga practice. They comprise nine simple stretches, a horizontal, diagonal and vertical set (see pp.40-7) which give your torso an all-round stretch and tone up your body in preparation for the rest of the postures. You follow these with two to three minutes of relaxation in a lying-down posture, the Corpse Pose (see p.52). Then you sit up and do two breathing exercises, followed by a simple meditation. The whole sequence takes a little over half an hour. You can practise it in the morning, ideally before breakfast, and in the evening, half an hour before eating, or two hours after an early evening meal.

Throughout your practice, you should bear the following in mind:

Never force yourself into any position or hold it for longer than feels comfortable. Remember, the yogic way is not a competition, even with yourself. Pain is a warning! When doing the exercises, be aware of your own flexibility and fitness. Slow and steady effort brings lasting results.

Always breathe in and out through your nostrils and do not exhale through your mouth. This will give you better breath control, and conserve energy, or prana.

Co-ordinate your breathing with your movements, and remain in each posture for about five seconds, either holding your breath after inhaling, or breathing normally after exhaling.

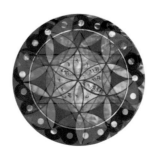

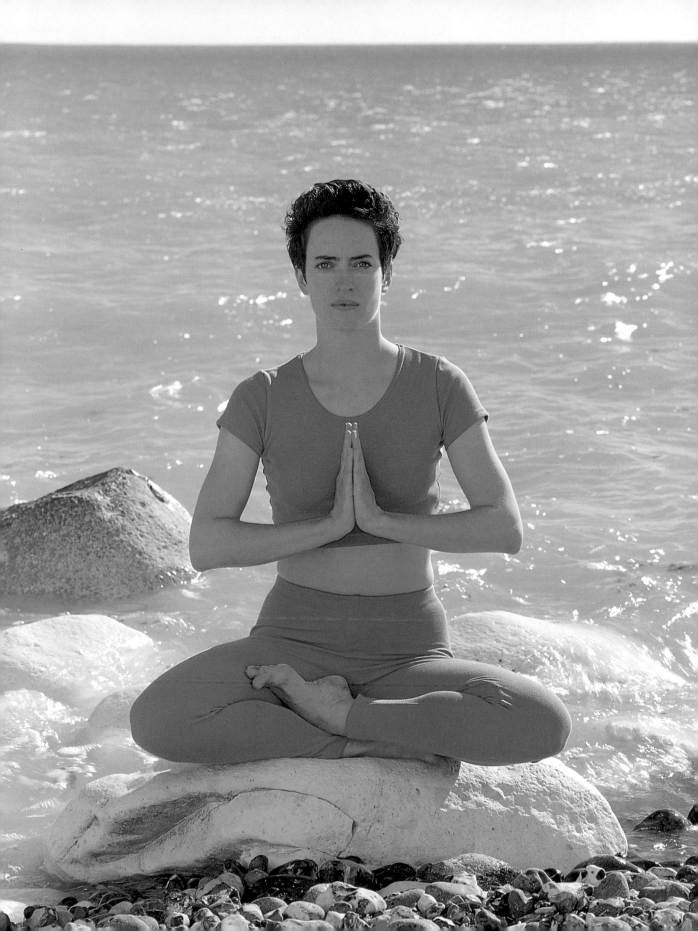

STRESS-RELIEVING STRETCHES

One of the main areas where physical tension accumulates is in the middle of your shoulders and at the nape of your neck. By contracting and stretching these areas, you can release tension throughout your whole body. Practise nine postures, in sets of three, as set out on these pages (pp.40-7). Each set consists of a vertical, horizontal and diagonal stretch, and contraction to make sure that you exercise the whole of your torso.

In the first week, practise the vertical and horizontal stretches three times each, and the diagonal stretches twice on each side. From the second week onward, practise them four and three times each, respectively.

CAUTION

If you are a beginner, or if you have any difficulty getting into the Half-Lotus, do not attempt it. Sit in a simple cross-legged position instead. Remember to keep your back straight.

Vertical Stretch I - *one*

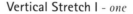

To get into the Half-Lotus, bend your right knee and bring the foot in placing it high on your left thigh. Bend your left knee, bring the left foot in and put it under your right thigh. Otherwise sit in any comfortable position, with your back, shoulders and neck straight, but without being rigid. Keep your arms loose by your sides. Loosen up your shoulders and arms by rolling them slowly.

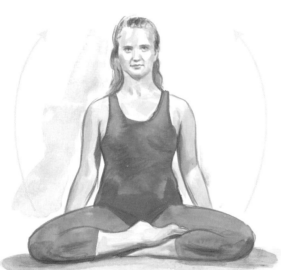

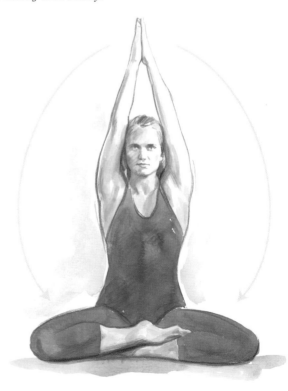

Vertical Stretch I - *two*

With your palms facing up, slowly raise your arms, inhaling. Press your palms together above your head, with your thumbs crossed. Keep stretching up. Hold for five seconds, retaining your breath. Slowly lower your arms, exhaling. Repeat three times. Loosen up.

Horizontal Stretch I - *one*

Stretch your arms forward, at shoulder height, palms together, thumbs crossed, with your chin pressed against your chest. Hold your back straight. Keep stretching your arms forward, breathing normally.

CAUTION

When practising the following shoulder and neck stretches (see pp.40-51), in all back bending movements, only go as far back as feels comfortable. Be careful not to strain yourself.

Horizontal Stretch I - *two*

Inhaling, move your arms apart and backward, looking upward. Hold your breath for five seconds, feeling the contraction of your shoulder and neck muscles.

Horizontal Stretch I - *three*

Move your arms forward, exhaling. Bend your head forward, press your chin into your chest, while keeping your back straight. Repeat twice more, and then loosen up.

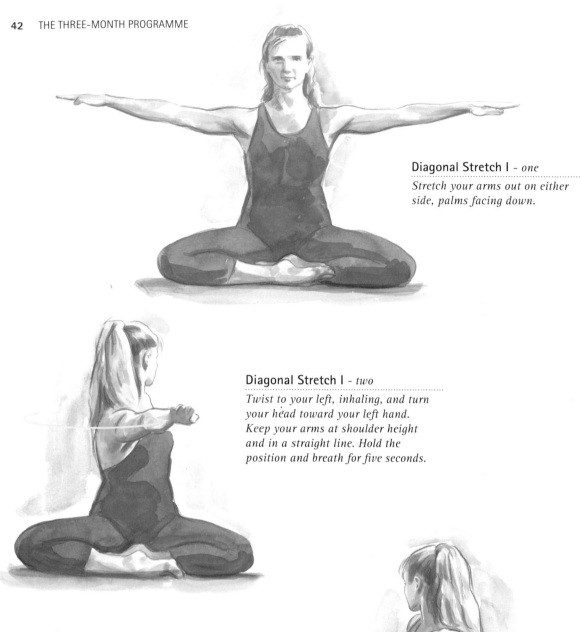

Diagonal Stretch I - *one*
Stretch your arms out on either side, palms facing down.

Diagonal Stretch I - *two*
Twist to your left, inhaling, and turn your head toward your left hand. Keep your arms at shoulder height and in a straight line. Hold the position and breath for five seconds.

Diagonal Stretch I - *three*
Exhaling, twist to the right in the same way, looking toward your right hand, and breathe for five seconds. Then twist to the left, inhaling as you did in step two. Repeat twice on each side. Face forward, inhaling, and lower your arms, exhaling. You should loosen up between each step.

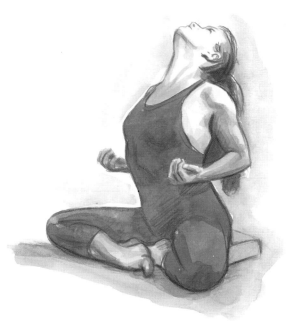

Horizontal Stretch II - *one*

Sit upright in a comfortable position, elbows by your sides and forearms parallel to the floor. Breathe normally. Move your elbows backward, inhaling, moving your head back. Hold your breath for five seconds, closing your elbows, so that you can feel the centre of your shoulders and neck contracting.

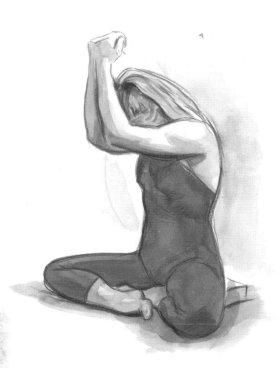

USEFUL TIPS

Keep these points in mind:
Try to set a regular time for your practice, either before breakfast, or two hours after a light meal.

....

If you wish to take a shower afterwards, wait for 15 minutes before doing so.

....

Never push yourself beyond your limits.
You can pull a muscle only by forcing yourself beyond your capacity, or by doing a movement too quickly.

....

If you do hurt yourself, gently massage the area and stop the posture for the day. Massage a few times daily until the pain goes. Gently resume when you feel ready.

Horizontal Stretch II - *two*

Move your elbows forward, exhaling, until they are level with your shoulders. Place your chin on your chest, keeping your back straight, and try to bring your elbows together. Breathe for five seconds, feeling the stretch in your neck and shoulders. Repeat three times. Lower your arms and loosen up.

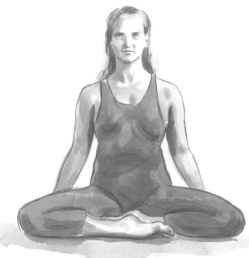

Vertical Stretch II

Sit cross-legged with your arms loose by your sides. Raise your shoulders, inhaling, and try to press the sides of your neck with your shoulders. Hold your breath in this position for five seconds, then slowly lower your shoulders, exhaling. Repeat three times. Then loosen up.

If you are a beginner you can hold your breath for a few seconds after inhaling, but never hold your breath out after exhaling.

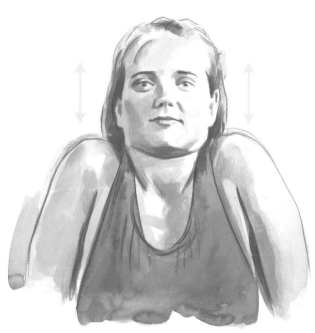

USEFUL TIPS

You should apply this advice to the whole of your practice:

Breathe out on a forward movement, or when you bend forward.

....

Breathe in on a backward movement, or when you stretch backward.

....

Breathe steadily when holding a posture.

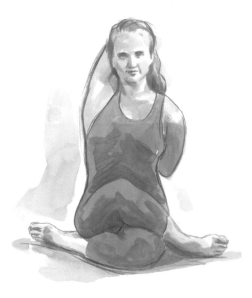

Diagonal Stretch II - *one*

*Sit in any comfortable cross-legged position.
You could try the Gomukhasana Pose (see
left). Bend your left knee and place your left
heel by the side of your right hip, then
moving your right leg over your left thigh,
try to align your two knees, and then place
your right heel by the side of your left hip.
Raise your right elbow and lower your left
elbow, trying to let your fingers touch
behind your back (if possible interlocking).*

Diagonal Stretch II - *two*

*Twist to the left, as far as you can,
inhaling, and look to your left
shoulder. Hold the position and
your breath for five seconds.*

Diagonal Stretch II - *three*

*Twist to the right, exhaling, and look
to your right elbow, breathing for five
seconds. Do this twice on each side.
Then face forward, inhaling, and lower
both hands, exhaling. Loosen up your
wrists, forearms, elbows and shoulders.*

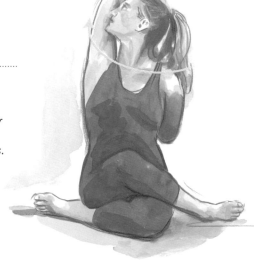

Vertical Stretch III - *one*

*Raise your arms and clasp
the fingers of both hands to get
a good grip. Stretch up while
inhaling, and hold your breath
for five seconds.*

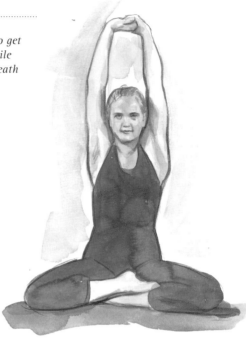

Vertical Stretch III - *two*

*Pulling your fingers, bend
your elbows and bring your
clasped hands back behind
your head, exhaling. Breathe
for five seconds, pushing your
elbows back to feel your
shoulder muscles contracting
and your chest stretching.
Repeat three times.*

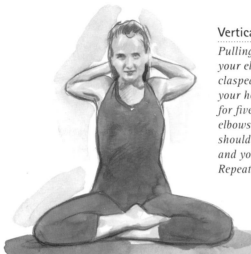

Horizontal Stretch III - *one*

*You should practise this stretch
three times.
    Bring your arms forward level
with your shoulders, fingers
clasped. Press your chin into your
chest to give the neck muscles a
good stretch. Stretch your arms
forward, inhaling, and hold the
breath for five seconds.*

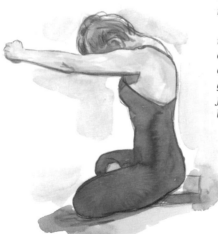

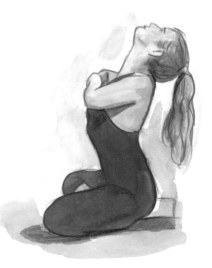

Horizontal Stretch III - *two*

*With your fingers clasped, bend your elbows,
bring your fists back to your chest, exhaling,
and bend your head back. Breathe for five
seconds, pushing your shoulders back, feeling the muscles contract in the neck and the
middle of the shoulders. Repeat step one.*

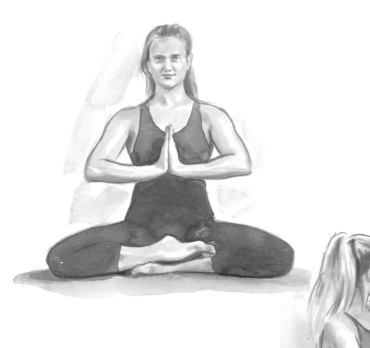

Diagonal Stretch III

Press your palms together against your chest, elbows parallel to the floor. Twist to the left, inhaling, and look to your left shoulder. Hold your breath for five seconds. Twist to the right, exhaling, and look to your right shoulder. Breathe for five seconds. Repeat twice on each side. Face forward, inhaling. Lower your arms, exhaling and loosen up.

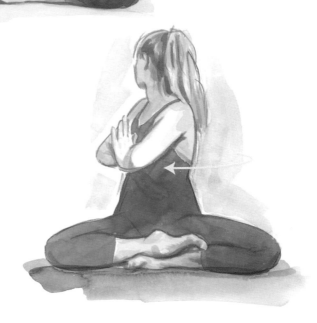

USEFUL TIPS

When practising these stretches and the other *asanas* remember these tips:

Do not swing from one posture to another without pausing for 5 seconds between postures.

....

Having twisted to the left or to the right, in each position, squeeze a little further in the same direction, while holding the breath or breathing freely.

....

Begin and end vertical and horizontal movements with your arms in a stretched position.

....

If you experience cramp, stop immediately, and gently massage the area until the discomfort goes, then start again.

NECK MOVEMENTS

You can practise a combination of neck movements to help relieve stress. When you feel stress accumulating in the neck and shoulder muscles, try these stretches.

After doing the first series of stretches involving the upper part of the body (see pp.40-7), you can follow these with four neck stretches (see pp.48-51).

When you are under stress, your breath will be shallow. However, by breathing deeply with each movement, you will train your lungs to breathe properly.

CAUTION

If you have arthritis of the cervical spine, or rheumatoid arthritis, only practise the neck movements under the guidance of a yoga therapist.

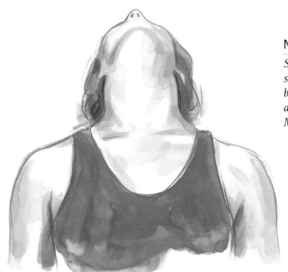

Neck Stretch I - *one*

Sit in a comfortable position, with your shoulders and back straight, arms loose by your sides. Loosen up your shoulders and neck muscles. Breathe normally. Move your head backward, inhaling.

Neck Stretch I - *two*

Move your head all the way forward (without bending your body forward), exhaling, until your chin is pressed into your chest. Keep your shoulders relaxed. Repeat two to three times. Then lift your head up, inhaling. Exhale and loosen up.

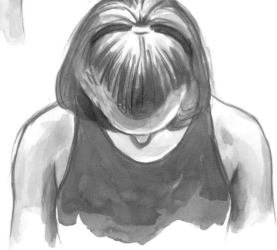

Neck Stretch II

Face forward. Turn your head to the left as far as you can, inhaling, then all the way to the right, exhaling. Repeat two to three times on each side, each movement taking about five seconds. Then face forward, inhaling. Exhale and loosen up.

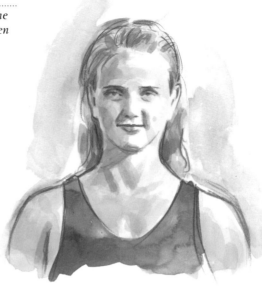

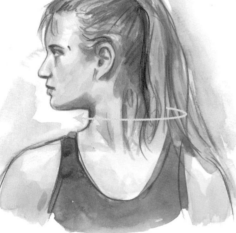

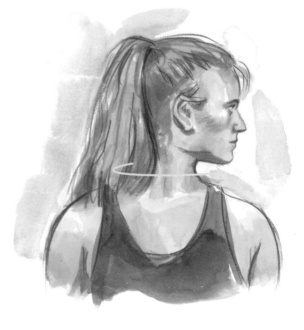

USEFUL TIPS

Whenever practising the *asanas* and breathing exercises bear the following in mind:

Always wear loose and comfortable clothing.

....

Keep your eyes closed to maintain inner calm.

....

If you wear glasses, take them off.

....

Loosen up before, in between and after each exercise.

Neck Stretch III - *one*

Face forward. Inhale deeply. Bend your head down to your left shoulder, exhaling, without turning your head or lifting your left shoulder. Lift your head up, inhaling, and lower your head to your right, exhaling. Repeat two to three times on each side. Lift your head up, inhaling, and exhale. Loosen up.

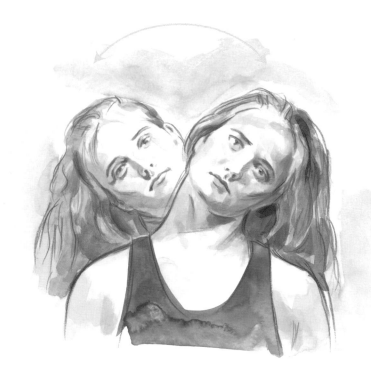

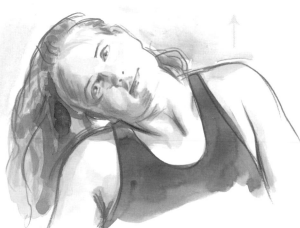

Neck Stretch III - *two*

Do the same movements as in step one, but when bending your head to the left, lift your right shoulder up and bring it as close to the side of your neck as you can, while keeping your left shoulder straight. Repeat on the other side.

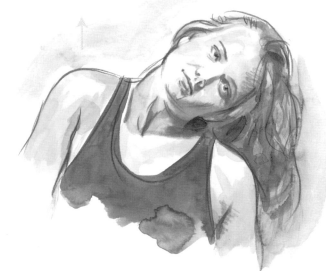

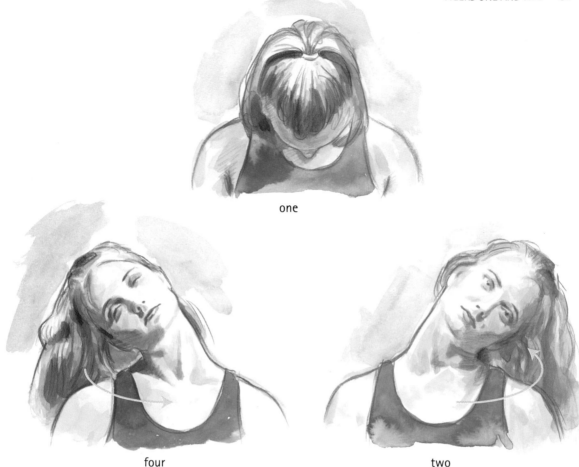

one

four

two

Neck Roll

Face forward. Inhale deeply. Exhaling, bend your head forward until your chin is pressed into your chest. Move your head gently, in a circular motion from the left, inhaling, until your head tilts backward. Then continue to roll your head in the same direction, exhaling, until your chin is pressed into your chest again. Stretch gently before lifting your head up, inhaling, and exhale. Inhale again, lower your head, exhaling, and press your chin into your chest. Repeat the sequence in the opposite direction. Then repeat twice in each direction. Loosen up.

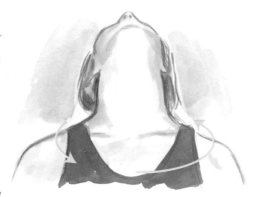

three

BREATHING EXERCISES

For the past three thousand years, yogis have prepared the mind for meditation by practising deep and slow breathing. *Pranayama* is the science of breath control. *Prana* means "breath" and *ayama*, "lengthening". By learning to breathe correctly, you can release tension and calm the mind.

There are two specific breathing exercises which you can practise regularly to help relieve and prevent stress. They are *Nadi-Sodhana*, or Alternate-Nostril Breathing, and *Ujjayi*, or breathing through both nostrils while gently contracting the muscles inside the throat.

Do the two exercises on their own, first *Nadi-Sodhana* and then *Ujjayi*, or after the first series of stretches, having relaxed for three minutes in *Shavasana* (the Corpse Pose, see below).

Shavasana is the classic relaxation pose. Practise it between the different sequences for at least three minutes. After a full session of yoga, relax in it for ten to fifteen minutes, by which time your mind should be completely calm and absorbed in peace.

DEEP BREATHING

When you are under stress, deep breathing helps to release tension. So, whenever you feel tense, inhale deeply, letting your abdomen expand gently, and exhale slowly, letting it contract. This is how you breathe naturally. Do not lift your chest while inhaling. Breathe deeply half a dozen times, in and out. Then breathe naturally for a minute. Repeat the cycle.

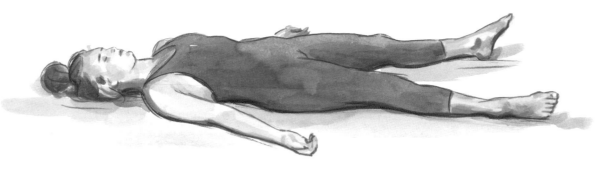

USEFUL TIPS

Before practising *pranayama* clean your nostrils to clear out any mucus.

....

Before starting, empty your bladder and bowels.

....

Practise *pranayama* a couple of hours after eating, or else before a meal.

....

Wear a sweater or a shawl if the room temperature falls below 22°C (72°F).

....

When doing *pranayama*, keep your eyes closed.

....

After the last exercise, sit still for at least two minutes, breathing normally.

The Corpse Pose – Shavasana

Lie down on your back, arms by your sides, palms facing up, legs slightly apart, and your eyes closed. Breathe through your nostrils, allowing the breath to flow in rhythm with your lungs. Feel peaceful and at rest. Consciously relax your whole body. When you practise this for a short while, your consciousness will start to flow gently throughout your body. Imagine a sense of wellbeing throughout, the prana, *or the vital force, softly coursing through it, revitalising the cells, and the internal organs.*

ALTERNATE-NOSTRIL BREATHING

Nadi-Sodhana means purification (*sodhana*) of the nerve currents (*nadis*). The *nadis* are metaphorical nerve channels in the energy body through which *prana*, or the vital energy, flows.

The purpose of this breathing exercise is to counteract physical and mental tension. By regulating the breath, and deepening and lengthening it, you release tension from the *nadis,* calm the mind, and you feel relaxed.

The left nostril (the passive side), is the path of the *nadi* called *Ida*, the right nostril (the dynamic side), that of *Pingala*. The way in which they interact, with the flow of the two currents shifting from one nostril to the other, is reflected in the breath. In a state of physical and mental tension your breath will be shallow and spasmodic, whereas when your mind is calm and your body relaxed, the flow of the breath will be smooth and even.

The Nadi-Sodhana Mudra

In Nadi-Sodhana *you adopt a particular hand position or* Mudra.

Place your index and middle fingers in the middle of your forehead, between the eyebrows. Place your thumb on your right nostril and your ring and little finger on your left nostril.

In this Mudra *each finger has a special significance. The thumb represents the cultivation of will power, the index finger the "I", or oneself and the middle finger, the Absolute or one's spiritual being, the ring finger emotional maturity and the little finger control of the mind. The juxtaposition of the middle and index fingers symbolises the union of oneself with the Absolute or pure consciousness.*

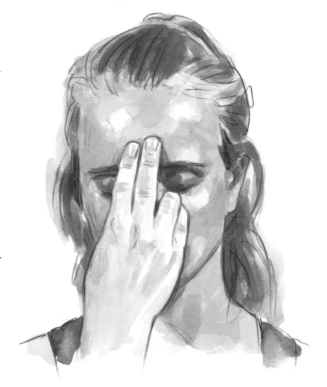

One round of Nadi–Sodhana

Sit comfortably, if you wish in the Easy Pose (see p.87). Adopt the following hand position (see p.53). Place the middle and index fingers in the centre of your forehead, between the eyebrows. Gently press the side of your right nostril with your right thumb. Rest the tip of your ring and little fingers lightly on the side of your left nostril. Inhale deeply through your left nostril, feeling the coolness of your breath in the nerves in the upper nostril and still further up inside your head.

Press your left nostril, lift your thumb from the right, and exhale slowly and fully, feeling the warmth of the breath inside the right nostril. Inhale through the right nostril, feeling the coolness as before, and exhale through the left, feeling the warmth. Repeat for five rounds, making a total of six. Lower your hand and breathe naturally for a minute.

You inhale slowly and deeply, and exhale slowly and fully, emphasising the outbreath.

CAUTION

Strictly avoid retaining the breath if you suffer from high blood pressure or epilepsy. Similarly for stress management, do not retain the breath, as this can build up tension.

VICTORIOUS BREATH - UJJAYI

Ujjayi is the second-most effective *pranayama* for stress relief. The term means mastery (*jaya*) in raising the energy level (*ud*). When tense, you may instinctively gulp air, in the hope that this will alleviate tension. You can use this *pranayama* to release tension in the solar plexus or abdomen.

Ujjayi is a body-warming *pranayama* and helps to eliminate phlegm. It also strengthens the nervous and digestive systems.

This *pranayama* quietens the mind and lessens anxiety. It is simple to do and has a naturally calming effect even after only two or three minutes practice. By breathing in and out through a slightly constricted glottis, the breath becomes naturally long and slow without effort.

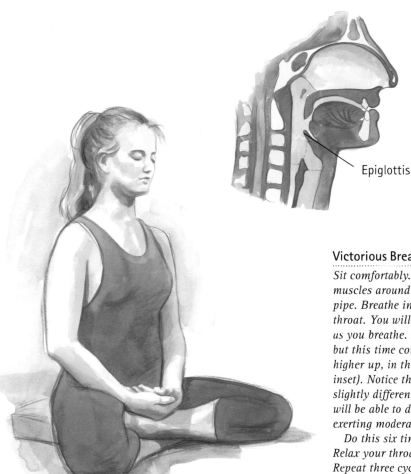

Epiglottis

Victorious Breath

Sit comfortably. Contract the glottis, or the muscles around the opening of your wind-pipe. Breathe in deeply. Focus on your throat. You will hear a slight hissing sound as you breathe. Exhale as slowly as you can, but this time contract the muscles a little higher up, in the area of the epiglottis (see inset). Notice that your breath now sounds slightly different. With enough practice you will be able to do this contraction well, exerting moderate pressure.

Do this six times, breathing in and out. Relax your throat and breathe for a while. Repeat three cycles, to make a total of four.

MEDITATION ON PEACE & FREEDOM

In meditation you aim to reach a state where you are aware of
an inner peace, and experience a sense of release from everything
impeding that peace. Meditation does not mean contemplation
alone; it is also a healing process. The word "meditation" derives
from the Latin, *mederi*, to heal. It means to heal a mental affliction
caused by psychological stress, firstly by achieving an inner calm
and then, in a peaceful state of mind, contemplating the problem,
its cause and how to resolve it.

In the first fortnight of the Three-Month Programme, you can
learn this basic meditation practice, which you can do as the third
part of the opening sequence, beginning with the nine stretches
(see pp.40-7), and the two breathing exercises (see pp.52-5).

You can practise this meditation after the stretches and
breathing exercises, either before breakfast or following the day's
activities, ideally, twice a day. Or you can practise it on its own,
at another time, and for longer if you like.

After practising
Nadi-Sodhana and *Ujjayi
pranayamas* (see pp.53-5) and
sitting relaxed for a couple of
minutes, loosen up your shoulders, neck
and legs. Resume the Easy Pose (see p.87).
If you prefer a chair, choose one which is
neither too soft nor too hard, with a straight
back. Keep both your legs together, and the
weight of your feet equally distributed.

Place your hands in your lap, one on top of the other,
palms facing up, or on your knees, the tips of the index
finger and thumb together, palms either facing up or down.

Keep your eyes closed. Feel peaceful, and detached. Do not feel
the need to do anything. Breathe spontaneously. After a minute,
become aware of your breath, the coolness of the in-flow deep
inside your head, and the warmth of the out-flow inside your lower
nostrils. Train your mind to be more and more aware of the breath.

By concentrating on the flow of your breath, you will notice your
breathing automatically slowing down.

In a relaxed state of mind,
focus on *prana*, the vital energy of
the breath. Allow your thoughts to flow
undisturbed. Experience the alternating
coolness and warmth of the breath. After a couple
of minutes, associate your awareness of peace with
the feeling of coolness, and the release of inner
tension with the warmth.

Guide these two feelings by repeating mentally, from time to
time, "peace" inhaling, and "freedom" exhaling. Use these words
to guide the flow of a particular feeling, so that it suffuses your
consciousness. After a minute, pause and just be aware of the breath
for the next minute. Then resume the repetition slowly and clearly.
When thoughts persist in floating into your mind, repeat to yourself
"I am full of inner peace", inhaling, and "I am a free soul", exhaling.

Pause again, to be aware of the breath for a minute, and then resume the
repetition of "peace" and "freedom". In the last few minutes of this ten-minute
session, repeat "harmony, profound inner harmony", inhaling; then "all tension
is draining out", exhaling. "Gathering in the fullness of peace", inhaling;
"smoothing out all conflicts", exhaling. "Goodness, beauty, grace and poise flowing in",
inhaling; "pain, unhappiness, anxiety and stress flowing out", exhaling.

Detach your mind and relax for a couple of minutes before getting up.

USEFUL TIPS

Even if you are able to sit in the Lotus, it is not really
suitable for meditation because your legs may go to sleep
or start aching.

....

Find a posture which will allow you to sit still without
straining, or making too conscious an effort.

....

Keep your back and shoulders straight, so you can
breathe properly.

....

The more aware you are of the breath, the greater the
consciousness of peace and liberation will be in
your subconscious.

....

How far you experience the positive effects will depend on
your faith in the practice.

CHAPTER FOUR

Weeks three and four

In the third and fourth weeks, you can add nine additional stretches based on the lumbar region (the area between the lower ribs and hip bones) to your sessions. But first of all repeat the nine stretches involving the upper part of the body from weeks one and two (see pp.40-7), followed by the neck movements (see pp.48-51).

After the neck movements, rest for a couple of minutes in the Corpse Pose (see p.52), stretch your legs and loosen up. Relax your arms and shoulders.

Now begin the next series of lumbar stretches (see pp.60-9) which cover weeks three to four of the Three-Month Programme. The first place where tension tends to accumulate is in the middle of the shoulders, at the base of the neck. The second place where it builds up is in the lumbar region. So try the following nine postures as additional help for stress relief in these areas.

Due to poor posture we can easily strain the muscles and ligaments in the lumbar region. Many people experience low back pain for which there is no physical cause, and which is often a symptom of stress. These lumbar stretches are designed to relieve muscle spasm and alleviate the type of back discomfort which is caused by stress and tension.

Start with a backward followed by a forward bend. Backward bends are energising, whereas forward bends quieten the mind and body.

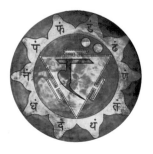

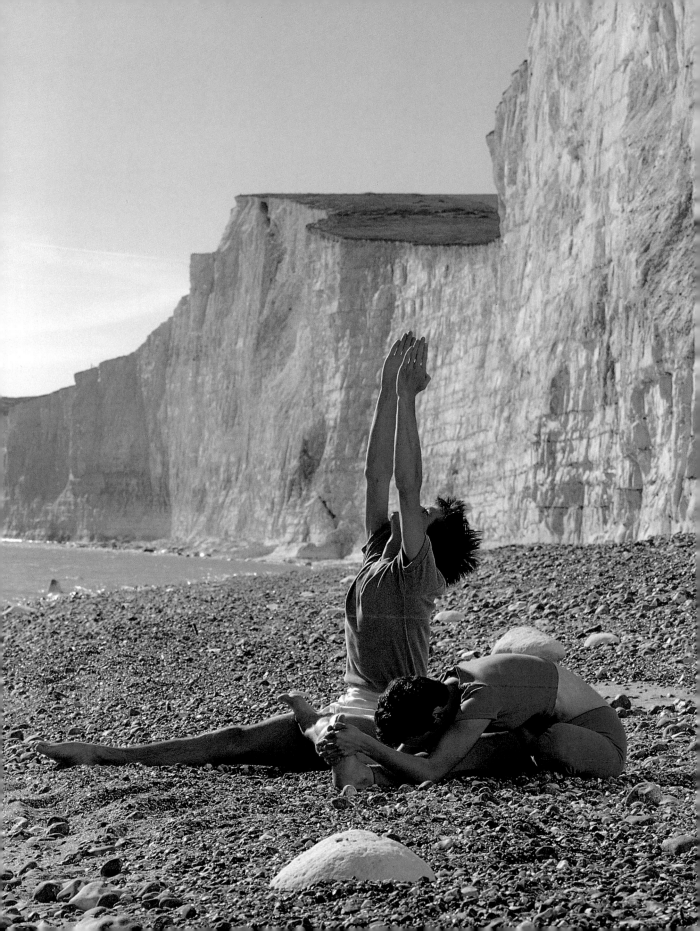

THE LUMBAR STRETCHES

When performing the forward-bending stretches, be careful to bend from the hips, and keep the breastbone stretching forward, thus stretching the lumbar region without rounding it. If your hip joints are stiff, straining to bring the trunk forward may damage the back, so be careful not to overdo the movement, and always move slowly.

In the backward-arching lumbar stretches you should lengthen the trunk from breastbone to pubis before you arch back, otherwise you may compress the backs of the lumbar vertebrae together.

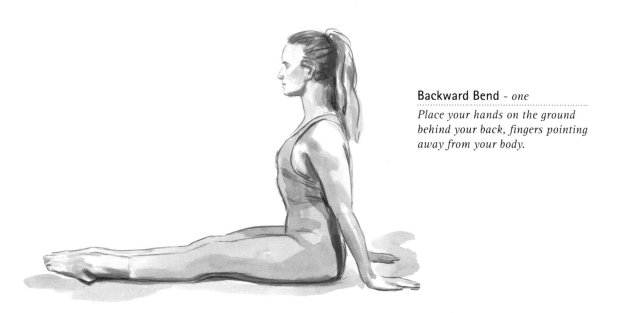

Backward Bend - *one*
Place your hands on the ground behind your back, fingers pointing away from your body.

Backward Bend - *two*
Lift your hips up, inhaling, tilt your head backward. Sit down slowly, exhaling. Repeat twice. Loosen your wrists, arms and legs.

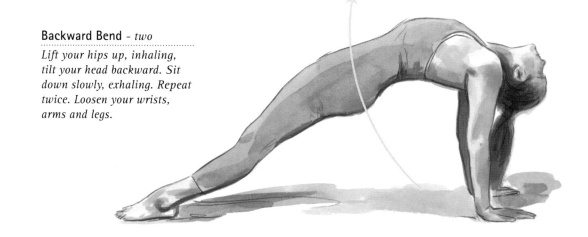

Lumbar Forward Bend - *one*

Bring your heels together, flexing the knees and ankles, soles apart. Place your arms between your legs and your hands under your ankles.

Lumbar Forward Bend - *two*

Stretch backward, inhaling, bending your head back and straightening your elbows. Hold your breath for five seconds.

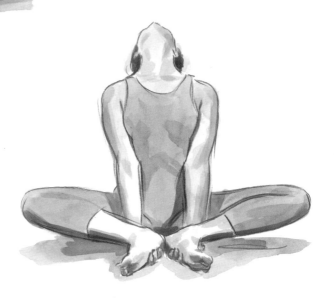

CAUTION

If you have bulging or prolapsed discs you should only do forward bends under the guidance of a yoga therapist trained in back care.

Lumbar Forward Bend - *three*

Bend forward, exhaling, lowering your elbows close to the ground, and your head as far down as you can, feeling the pull in your shoulders and the lumbar region. Breathe for 10 seconds. Repeat three times. Stretch your legs and loosen up.

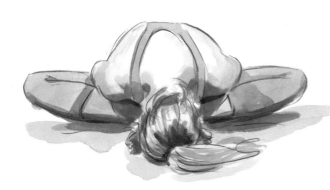

Sideways Bend - *one & two*

Bring the soles of your feet together, bending your knees as much as you can. Hold your feet with both hands. Inhale, bend to the left, exhaling, and moving your head to your right shoulder, look forward.

Bring your head up, inhaling, bend to the right, exhaling. Move your head to the left shoulder. Bring your head up, inhaling, and exhale. Repeat twice on each side. Stretch your legs and loosen up.

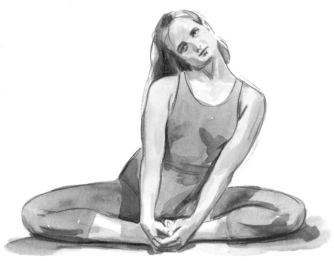

CAUTION

If you are a beginner, or if you have any difficulty getting into the Half-Lotus (see p.40), do not attempt it. Sit in a simple cross-legged position instead, taking care to keep your back straight.

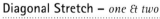

Diagonal Stretch – *one & two*

Sit cross-legged. Join your fingers behind your neck. Inhale, hold your breath and twist to the left.

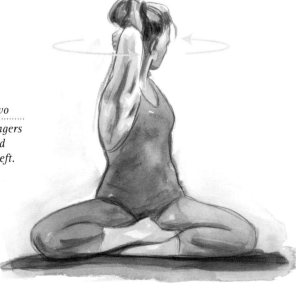

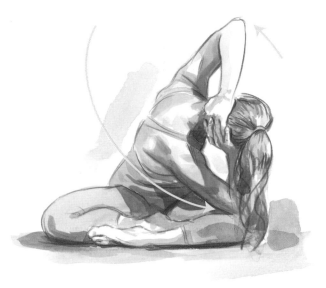

Diagonal Stretch - *three*

Bring your right elbow down to your left knee, exhaling, and lifting up the other elbow, look up to it. Sit up, inhaling, face forward. Hold your breath.

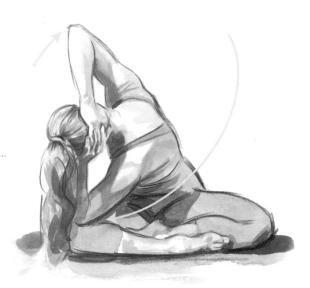

Diagonal Stretch - *four*

Twist to the right, bringing your left elbow down to your right knee, exhaling. Lift up your right elbow and look up at it.

Diagonal Stretch - *five*

Come up, inhaling, tilt your head backward.

Diagonal Stretch - *six*

Bend forward, exhaling and lower your head and elbows as close to the ground as possible. Sit up, inhaling, tilt your head backward. Lower your arms, face forward, exhaling. Repeat the movements, stretch your legs and loosen up.

Backward/Forward Bend - *one*

Place your left foot on top of your right thigh. If you find this difficult, place the sole against the inside of the thigh. Place your hands behind you on the floor, fingers pointing backward.

Backward/Forward Bend - *two*

Raise your hips, inhaling, tilt your head back. Sit down slowly, exhaling, arms by your sides.

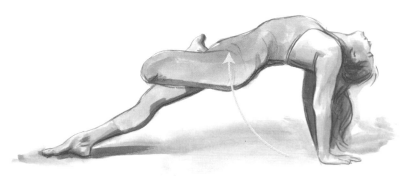

Backward/Forward Bend - *three*

Raise your arms above your head, inhaling. With your palms facing, lift your shoulders alternately a few times, looking up to your hands, and holding your breath for five seconds, to exercise the side muscles. Bend backward and stretch up.

Backward/Forward Bend - *four*

Bend forward on to your right leg, bringing your chest forward toward your foot, exhaling. Hold your feet or wherever you can reach with both hands. Breathe for 10 seconds, and point your toes toward your head to stretch the hamstring muscles. Repeat step three. Lower your arms, exhaling. Stretch your legs and loosen up. Repeat on the other side.

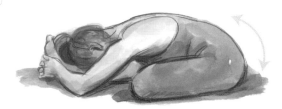

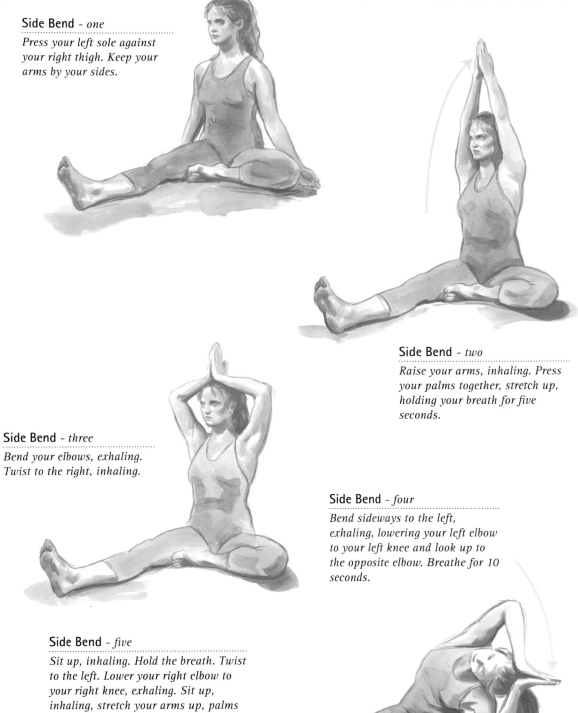

Side Bend - *one*

Press your left sole against your right thigh. Keep your arms by your sides.

Side Bend - *two*

Raise your arms, inhaling. Press your palms together, stretch up, holding your breath for five seconds.

Side Bend - *three*

Bend your elbows, exhaling. Twist to the right, inhaling.

Side Bend - *four*

Bend sideways to the left, exhaling, lowering your left elbow to your left knee and look up to the opposite elbow. Breathe for 10 seconds.

Side Bend - *five*

Sit up, inhaling. Hold the breath. Twist to the left. Lower your right elbow to your right knee, exhaling. Sit up, inhaling, stretch your arms up, palms together, holding your breath. Lower your arms, exhaling. Repeat on the other side.

Diagonal Bend - *one*

Stretch your legs out in front of you, keeping them together. Join the tips of your thumbs and place your palms down on the ground by the side of your left hip. Bend your head back, inhaling and hold your breath for five seconds.

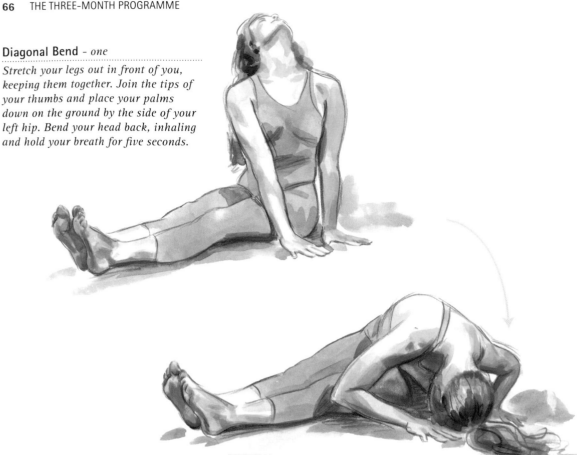

Diagonal Bend - *two*

Bend down, exhaling. Slide your hands forward a little, so that you can place your forehead on the floor between them.

Diagonal Bend - *three*

Sit up, inhaling. Lower your right hip to the ground, sliding your hands slightly forward and bending your head back. Hold your breath. Repeat once more. Then, sitting up in the same way, face forward and exhale. Loosen up before carrying out the same movements twice on the other side.

Pelvic Bend - *one*

Place your left foot on top of your right thigh. If you find this difficult, place the left sole against the inside of the thigh. Place both hands on top of your left knee. Pressing the knee down, bend your head back, inhaling.

Pelvic Bend – *two*

Lift your knee up, pressing your thigh against the left side of your abdomen and chest, and lower your forehead to your knee, exhaling. Breathe for 10 seconds. Lower the knee down, bending your head back, inhaling, as in step one.

Pelvic Bend - *three*

Raise your knee to your shoulder as before, place your left ear on your knee, exhaling, and breathe for 10 seconds. Lower your knee, bending your head back, inhaling. Stretch your legs and loosen up. Repeat on the other side.

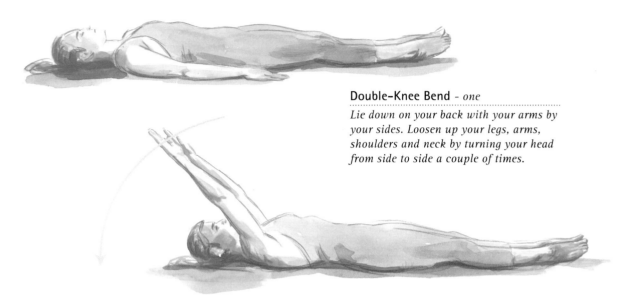

Double-Knee Bend - *one*

Lie down on your back with your arms by your sides. Loosen up your legs, arms, shoulders and neck by turning your head from side to side a couple of times.

Double-Knee Bend - *two*

Bring your legs together. Move your arms backward, inhaling, and hold your breath.

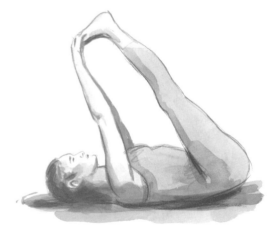

Double-Knee Bend - *three*

Holding your breath, raise both your arms and legs to the vertical position. Hold your legs wherever you can, if possible at the ankles or toes. If your back is weak, raise your legs with your knees slightly bent.

Double-Knee Bend - *four*

Exhaling, bend your knees to your chest and, pressing your knees with both hands, lift your head up. Keep your shoulders relaxed. With your forehead on, or close to your knees, breathe for 10 seconds.

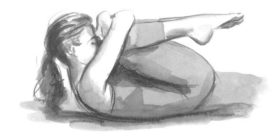

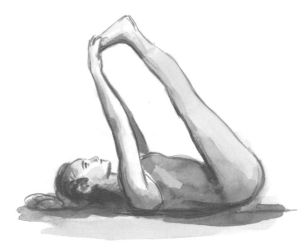

Double-Knee Bend - *five*

Inhaling, raise your arms and legs to the vertical position, and lower your head to the ground, holding your legs, as in step three. Keep your shoulders relaxed. Hold your breath for five seconds. Repeat twice. Stretching up your arms and legs, inhale. Hold your breath, with your head on the ground and hands on your legs. Then lower your legs and place your arms by the side of your head, exhaling.

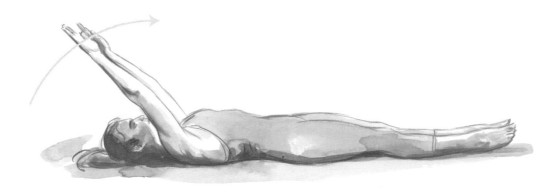

Double-Knee Bend - *six*

Bring your arms forward by your sides.

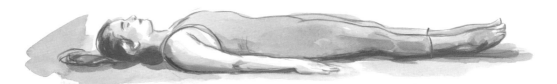

Once you have relaxed, sit up in a comfortable position, and do *Nadi-Sodhana* and *Ujjayi pranayamas* (see pp.53-5). Conclude the session by meditating on "peace" and "freedom" (see pp.56-7).

Double-Knee Bend - *seven*

Loosen up your shoulders and your legs. Move your hips to the left and to the right. Raise your hips gently up and down. Turn your head to the left and right a couple of times. Then rest for five minutes in the Corpse Pose (see p.52).

CHAPTER FIVE

Weeks five and six

In the fifth week, after having done the nine stretches based on the upper part of the body, from weeks one and two (see pp.40-7), relax in the Corpse Pose (see p.52) for three minutes, in preparation for the Shoulderstand (see pp.72-7).

The Shoulderstand is an inverted posture which can be of great benefit if you practise it with care. It helps to encourage circulation, improving the drainage of the veins and the lymphatic channels in the legs. The blood returning to the heart from the legs normally has to be carried against gravity, and this can strain the superficial veins, so that they become swollen and convoluted – "varicose veins". Such veins can be quite painful, especially if you have been standing for some time. Inversion of the body temporarily relieves the pressure and allows the veins to rest. In the same way lymph fluid is helped to drain away from the tissues round the feet, where it can otherwise accumulate in puffy, swollen ankles. Inversion helps the fluid to drain back toward the trunk via the small lymphatic channels, which run in parallel with the veins. The lymph eventually is returned to the blood stream.

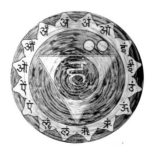

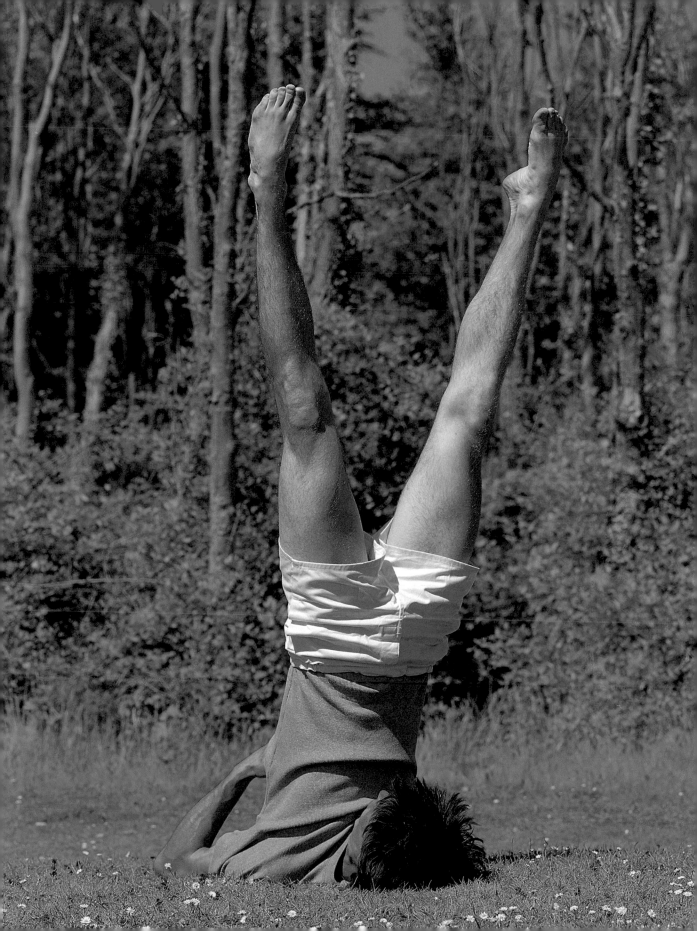

SHOULDERSTAND SERIES - SARVANGASANA

The Shoulderstand invigorates and rejuvenates your whole body, and is one of the most important postures for stress relief. The Sanskrit word *sarva* means entire or whole, and *anga*, limbs or parts. It is particularly beneficial for the thyroid gland, which plays an important role in keeping the endocrine (hormonal) system in balance. A healthy thyroid gland is vital for wellbeing. If you are under emotional stress, this will have an adverse effect on your thyroid gland.

If you are a beginner you should only spend one to two minutes in the Shoulderstand. Instead of attempting the whole sequence, practise only steps one to six, and then fourteen to nineteen to come out of the posture.

> **USEFUL TIPS**
> If you have a weak lower back, while coming up into the Shoulderstand, raise your legs with your knees bent. Otherwise, keep your legs straight. Come down very slowly, supporting your back with your hands.

Shoulderstand - *one*
Before beginning, warm up your shoulder and neck muscles. Lie on your back. Loosen your shoulders. Keeping your head on the ground, lift your chest gently up and down.

Shoulderstand - *two*
Place your palms under your neck, lift your head up, place your chin on your chest, and bring your elbows together.

Shoulderstand - *three*
Lower your head. Bring your arms forward by your sides. Move your shoulders and your head to the left and right. Relax your legs.

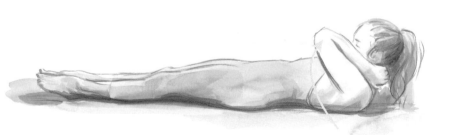

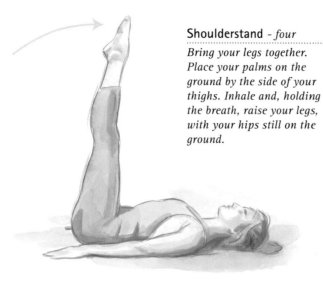

Shoulderstand - *four*

Bring your legs together. Place your palms on the ground by the side of your thighs. Inhale and, holding the breath, raise your legs, with your hips still on the ground.

Shoulderstand - *five*

Raise your hips, with your arms still on the ground.

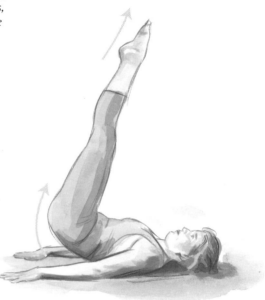

Shoulderstand - *six*

Straighten up, place your hands on your back, and exhale. Breathe for one to three minutes. Relax your legs and flex your ankles a few times. Press your chin into your chest.

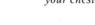

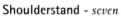

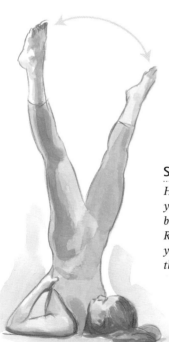

Shoulderstand - *seven*

Hold your back firmly. Move your legs apart, inhaling, and bring them together, exhaling. Repeat twice. This relaxes your leg muscles and helps the blood to flow downward.

Shoulderstand - *eight*

Bring your legs together. Inhale. Bend your left knee down to your left shoulder, exhaling. Straighten your leg up, inhaling. Repeat with the right knee.

USEFUL TIPS

If you spend a long time on your feet, or sitting down, you can practise steps eight and nine to help relax your legs further.

Shoulderstand - *nine*

Inhale. Exhaling, bend your left knee down to your right shoulder. Inhaling, straighten the leg up. Then, bend the right knee down to the left shoulder.

If your lumbar spine is very flexible, for increased benefit, continue with steps ten to thirteen.

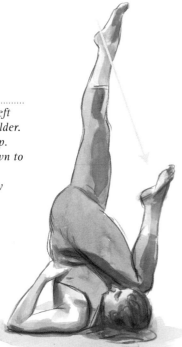

Shoulderstand - *ten*

Raise your legs straight up. Inhale. Hold your breath. Bend your legs, with your knees pointing up.

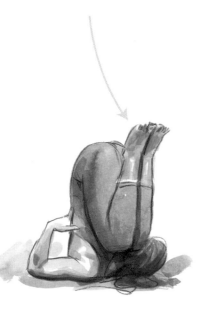

Shoulderstand - *eleven*

Twist to the left and lower both knees to the left shoulder, with the toes pointing up, exhaling. Lift your knees up, inhaling. Repeat on the right shoulder. After lifting your knees, straighten your legs, and breathe for 30 seconds.

Shoulderstand - *twelve*

Keep holding your back. Inhale. Exhale, lowering the left leg to the floor, behind your head, as far as you can, keeping the knee straight. Inhaling, raise your left leg. Repeat with the right leg.

USEFUL TIP:

By putting vertical and diagonal pressure on the abdomen, the movements in steps eight to thirteen will help to stimulate the colon, tone the large and small intestines, and relax the abdomen.

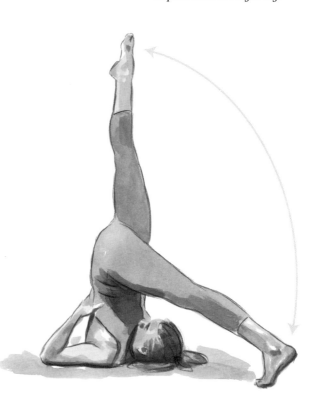

Shoulderstand - *thirteen*

Bring both legs straight down behind your head as far as you can, exhaling. Supporting your back with your hands, raise your legs up, inhaling. Breathe for 30 seconds.

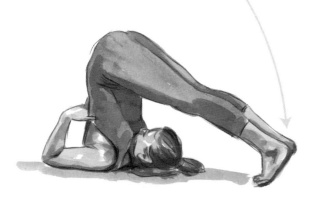

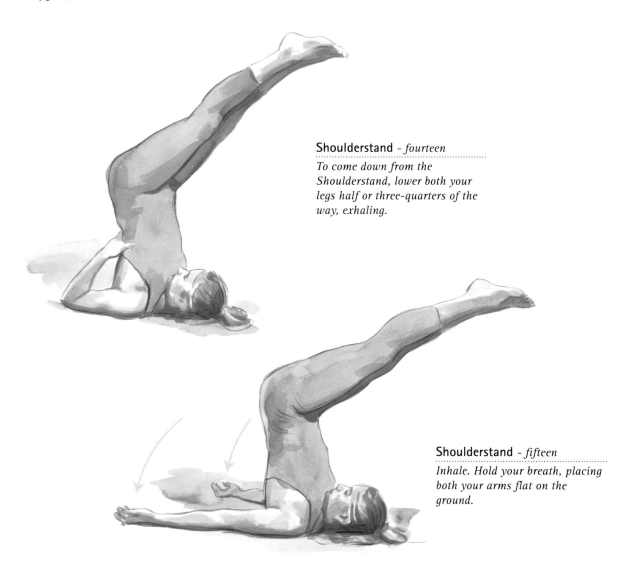

Shoulderstand - *fourteen*
To come down from the Shoulderstand, lower both your legs half or three-quarters of the way, exhaling.

Shoulderstand - *fifteen*
Inhale. Hold your breath, placing both your arms flat on the ground.

Shoulderstand - *sixteen*
Slowly lower your back and then your hips, keeping your head on the floor.

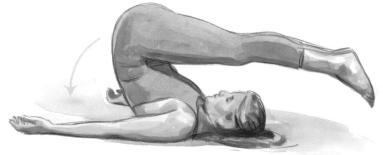

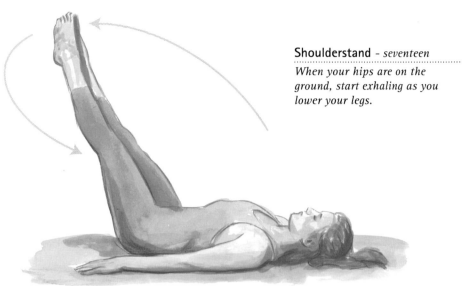

Shoulderstand - *seventeen*

When your hips are on the ground, start exhaling as you lower your legs.

Shoulderstand - *eighteen*

Bend both your knees on to your chest.

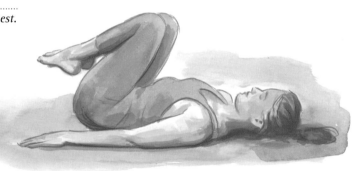

Shoulderstand - *nineteen*

Hold your knees, and rock your hips from side to side a few times. Place your feet on the ground and stretch your legs forward. Lift your hips gently up and down. Loosen up your legs. Rest in the Corpse Pose (see p.52) for two minutes.

USEFUL TIP
Afterwards it is important to loosen up your whole body, as in steps one to three (see p.72).

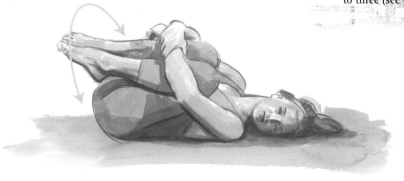

FISH POSE – MATSYASANA

The Fish Pose is the counterpose to the Shoulderstand, and should always be practised after it.

It is a backward bend for which you need strong back muscles to hold the lift of the upper back in the arched position. If you are a beginner, you should work on less strenuous backward bends, like the Bridge Pose (see pp.82-4), until you can hold the lift in the back without putting too much weight on your head.

By extending the ribcage fully, the Fish Pose helps you to breathe deeply and increases your lung capacity. By compressing the neck and upper spine it helps to release tension in the neck and shoulders. By giving a backward stretch to the lumbar spine, it removes stiffness and increases blood circulation to that area.

CAUTION

If your neck hurts, lower your shoulders and neck to the ground and loosen them up. Do not push yourself beyond your limits. Listen to your body.

Fish Pose - *one*

Lie relaxed with your legs together. Place your palms on the floor with the backs of your hands under your buttocks. Pressing your elbows down, lift your chest up and bend your head back, keeping the crown of your head on the floor. Breathe deeply for 30 seconds to one minute.

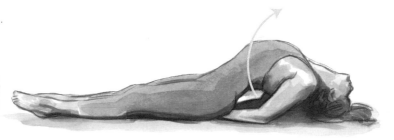

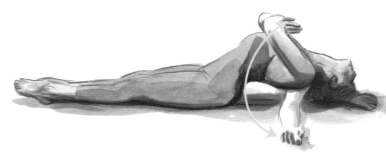

Fish Pose - *two*

If possible, bring your palms together on your chest.

Move your arms apart, inhaling, and bring your palms together, exhaling. Repeat once.

Fish Pose – *three*

Place your palms on your thighs.

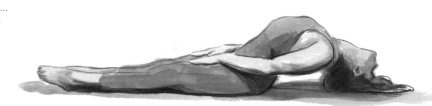

Fish Pose - *four*

Raise your arms, inhaling. Link your thumbs and bring them down above your head. Bring your arms forward, exhaling, and place your palms on your thighs. Repeat.

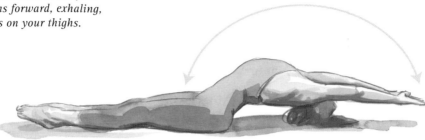

Fish Pose - *five*

Counterpose: Lower your neck and shoulders to the ground. Place your palms under your neck and lift your head up, keeping your chin on your chest. Bring your elbows together and breathe for five seconds in this position.

Fish Pose - *six*

Inhale first. Exhaling, bend your left knee to your left elbow, and stretch your right leg forward, inhaling. Keeping your head up, repeat on the other side.

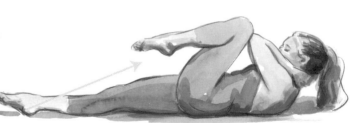

Fish Pose - *seven*

Inhale and keeping your head up, bend both knees to touch your elbows, exhaling. Stretch your legs forward, inhaling, and lower them to the floor. Lower your head. Bring your arms down by your sides and loosen up.

ALTERNATIVE FISH POSE - MATSYASANA

If you are very flexible, you can practise the following classical version of the Fish Pose on alternate days, instead of the basic posture for stress relief (see pp.78-9).

When practising the Fish Pose or its alternative, you should remain in the posture for at least half the time you stay in the Shoulderstand (see pp.72-7).

You can conclude the Alternative Fish Pose by doing three versions of *Yoga Mudra* (see p.81). *Yoga Mudra* helps the flow of *prana* or vital energy. It also relaxes the facial muscles, by increasing the blood flow to the face.

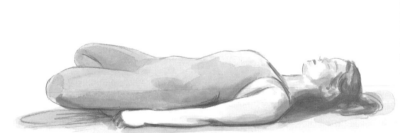

Alternative Fish Pose - *one*
Lie down. Bring your feet up under your thighs, crossing your legs. Hold your toes, and lower your knees to the ground. Pressing your elbows down, bend your head back, so that the top of your head rests on the floor. Breathe for a minute.

Alternative Fish Pose - *two*
With your palms together on your chest, do the same arm movements as in steps two and three in the basic pose (see p.78).

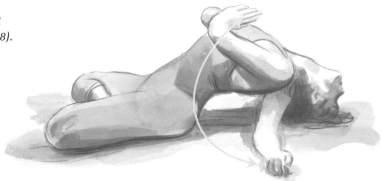

Alternative Fish Pose - *three*

Lower your neck and shoulders to the ground. Hold your elbows above your head. Breathe for 10 seconds. This releases tension from the shoulders and neck.

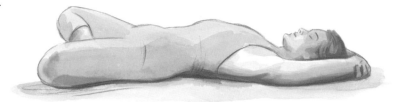

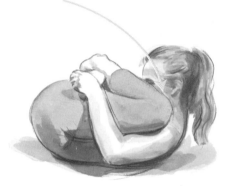

Alternative Fish Pose - *four*

With your legs crossed, hold your toes. Inhale. Bend your knees up to your shoulders, exhaling, and raise your head. In this position, inhale. Hold your breath, sit up and bend forward, exhaling. Breathe for five seconds. Conclude with Yoga Mudra.

Yoga Mudra - *one*

With your forehead on the floor, cross your fingers or grip them firmly behind your hips, and keep breathing for another five seconds.

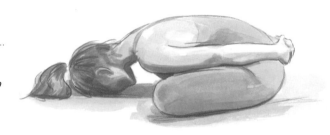

Yoga Mudra - *two*

Inhale. Gripping or crossing your fingers, raise your arms from your hips, as vertically as you can, breathing out fully. With your head on the ground, breathe for five seconds.

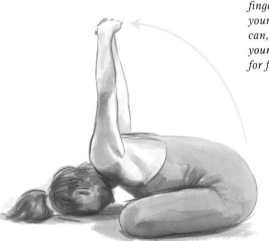

Yoga Mudra - *three*

Inhaling, bring your head backward, with your arms still raised and hold your breath. Then straighten up, exhaling. Lower your arms. Relax your shoulders. Turn your head from side to side. Stretch your legs out in front of you, and loosen up.

BRIDGE POSE – SETU BANDHASANA

After practising the Fish Pose (see pp.78-9), relax in the Corpse Pose (see p.52) for a couple of minutes before beginning the following variation of the Bridge Pose.

To complete the Shoulderstand series (see pp.72-7) you need to counterflex the cervical and lumbar spine. By raising your legs above your head in the Shoulderstand you bend the shoulders, neck and upper spine forward. In the Fish and the Bridge Pose you stretch the spine in the opposite direction.

By stretching the nerve centre in the solar plexus, this posture releases tension there, improving the digestion and helping to eliminate toxins from the abdomen. A tension-free solar plexus helps to calm the mind, just as psychological stress tenses up the nerves in the abdomen.

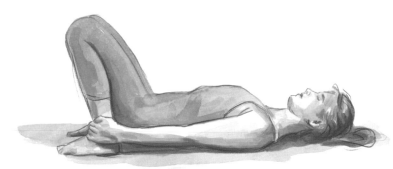

Bridge Pose - *one*

Lie down. Bend your knees and place your feet on the floor (a hip width apart) close to your buttocks. If you can, hold your ankles.

Bridge Pose - *two*

Lift your hips up as high as you can, inhaling, and lower them, exhaling.

USEFUL TIPS

If you are a beginner, omit steps three and four of the Bridge Pose.

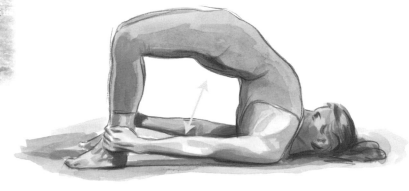

Bridge Pose - *three*

*Lift your hips up, inhaling, and exhale.
Hold your lower back firmly, supporting
your waist with your hands. Bring your
legs together and stretch them forward,
with the soles of your feet firmly on the
ground. Breathe for 10 seconds.*

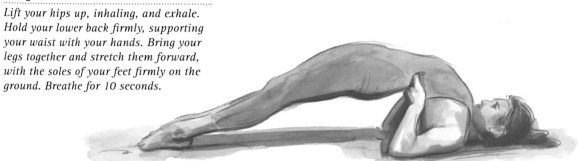

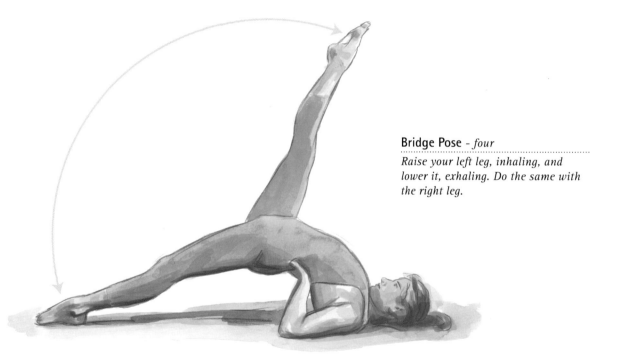

Bridge Pose - *four*

*Raise your left leg, inhaling, and
lower it, exhaling. Do the same with
the right leg.*

Bridge Pose - *five*

*To unwind from the Bridge Pose,
place your palms on top of your
thighs, and slowly stretch your legs
forward, lowering your hips to the
ground. Loosen up, and turn your
head from side to side.*

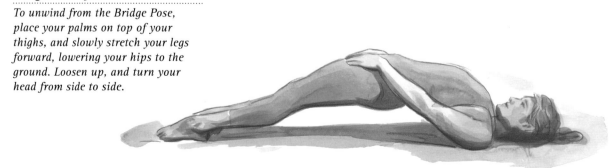

Additional Bridge Pose - *one*

*Bend your knees, with your feet
on the ground, close to your
buttocks. Place your palms on top
of your thighs.*

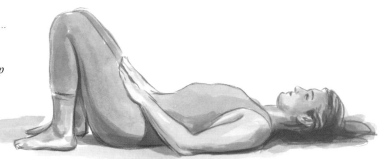

Additional Bridge Pose - *two*

*Raise your hips as high as you can,
moving your arms back and, linking
your thumbs, lower them above your
head, inhaling.*

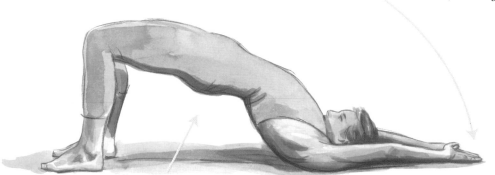

Additional Bridge Pose - *three*

*Lower your hips to the ground,
moving your arms forward, exhaling,
place your palms on top of your
thighs. Repeat twice. Stretch your legs
forward, arms by your sides, and
loosen up. Relax in the Corpse Pose
(see p.52) for a minute or two.*

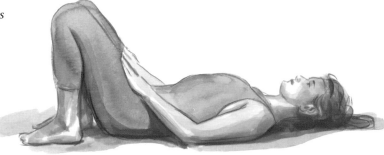

FORWARD BEND – PASCHIMOTTANASANA

Paschimottanasana, or the Forward Bend, means back (*paschima*) stretching (*uttana*). The back of the body is literally stretched from the heels to the top of the spine. This *asana* has many physical benefits, including stimulating the digestive organs, encouraging regular bowel movements and relieving constipation, regulating the working of the pancreas and massaging the abdominal organs.

You should begin this pose from the lying-down position to increase the effect on the back, chest and abdominal muscles. If, however, you have back problems, you should only do this from a sitting position.

> **USEFUL TIP**
> If you practise this together with the Abdominal Suction and Stretch (see below), these two exercises will have a very powerful effect on the abdominal organs, especially the pancreas.

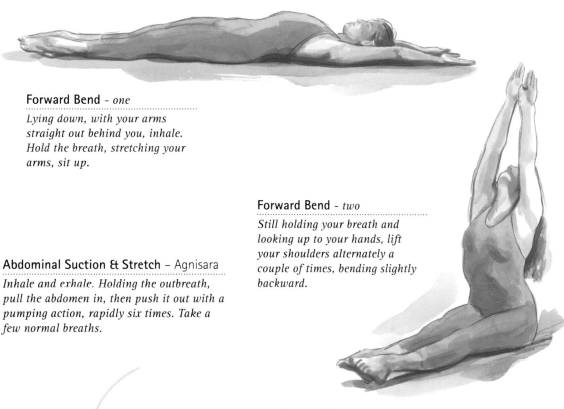

Forward Bend - *one*
Lying down, with your arms straight out behind you, inhale. Hold the breath, stretching your arms, sit up.

Forward Bend - *two*
Still holding your breath and looking up to your hands, lift your shoulders alternately a couple of times, bending slightly backward.

Abdominal Suction & Stretch – Agnisara
Inhale and exhale. Holding the outbreath, pull the abdomen in, then push it out with a pumping action, rapidly six times. Take a few normal breaths.

Forward Bend - *three*
Stretch up, and bend forward, exhaling. Hold your toes, or your ankles if possible. Point your toes toward your head, and breathe for 10 seconds. While holding this position you can do Agnisara (see above left). Raise your arms, inhaling, and stretch in the same way. Lower your arms, exhaling. Repeat once.

ADDITIONAL BREATHING EXERCISES

Sit in a comfortable posture, such as the Easy Pose/*Sukhasana* (see p.87), with your legs crossed, and your hands on your knees or in your lap. Breathe normally for a minute, then do the *Nadi-Sodhana* and *Ujjayi* breathing exercises (see pp.53-5). Breathe freely again for one minute before doing the following two *pranayamas*.

Both *Shitali* and *Shitakari* have a cooling effect on the body, relaxing the nerves and calming the mind.

Shitali

Curl up the sides of your tongue, letting the tip protrude slightly. Inhale slowly and deeply through the tip, concentrating on the coolness of the air flowing inside it. Close your mouth, pulling your tongue in, and exhale through your nose slowly and fully, with your mind relaxed.

Do this six times. Then breathe normally for a while, and repeat once more. Wait half a minute before going on to Shitakari.

USEFUL TIP

You should practise pranayama with your eyes closed, to maintain an inner calm. Do not forget to keep your back and shoulders straight.

Not everyone can curl up the sides of their tongue. Alternatively, keep your lips slightly apart and draw in air over the tip of the tongue.

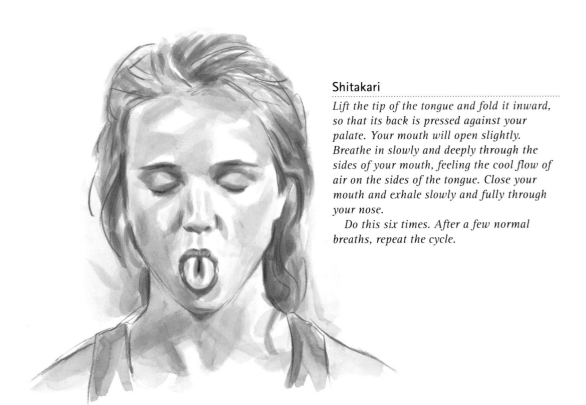

Shitakari

Lift the tip of the tongue and fold it inward, so that its back is pressed against your palate. Your mouth will open slightly. Breathe in slowly and deeply through the sides of your mouth, feeling the cool flow of air on the sides of the tongue. Close your mouth and exhale slowly and fully through your nose.

Do this six times. After a few normal breaths, repeat the cycle.

MEDITATION ON CONTENTMENT

You can conclude this fortnight with the fifteen minute meditation session which follows, or you can do it separately at a suitable time.

Following the same routine as in the preceding four weeks, meditate on "peace" and "freedom" for about eight minutes (see pp.56-7). Detach your mind, feel relaxed, and breathe normally for a minute.

Now be aware of the inflow and outflow of your breath, the coolness inside your head and the warmth within the lower nostrils. After a while, focus your attention only on the coolness, deep inside your head, and try to keep focusing on this awareness even when exhaling, and without concentrating on the warmth.

With each in-breath renew the feeling of coolness and imagine this sensation moving upward inside your head. From time to time, repeat "contentment", "deep contentment", "I am a contented soul". Absorb yourself in the meditation, trying to let go, allowing an inner harmony to fill your consciousness, as the feeling of coolness soars inside your head.

After about five minutes, detach your mind, breathe normally for a minute or two and, feeling relaxed, conclude the meditation.

Easy Pose - Sukhasana

When practising the meditation and breathing exercises you can sit cross-legged with your hands resting lightly on your knees, the tips of your index fingers touching your thumbs, or if you prefer with your hands in your lap. If you wish you can place a cushion under your buttocks for increased comfort.

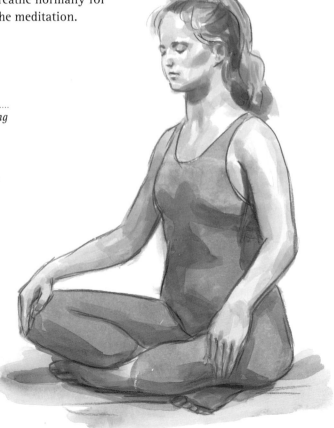

CHAPTER SIX

Weeks seven and eight

In weeks seven and eight, you can replace the Shoulderstand series (see pp.72-7) with the Cobra series (see pp.94-105). The Cobra series consists of three basic backward movements centred on the lumbar region, and three forward ones. As in the Shoulderstand series, you should do an inverted pose before the backward stretches.

Having done the nine basic stretches from weeks one and two (see pp.40-7), begin with the Bowing-Down Pose (see p.90), and then go into a semi-inverted posture, the Half-Headstand (see pp.91-2), and finish with a variation of the Dog Pose (see p.92).

Inverted and semi-inverted postures are very useful for releasing tension by improving the circulation of blood to the brain, and by making you breathe deeply, thus calming the mind. The increased blood flow aids general health and maintains hormonal balance, ensuring that the pituitary gland functions well. The Bowing-Down Pose, the Half-Headstand and the Dog Pose, all have a very powerful effect on the internal organs, in the same way as the Shoulderstand (see pp.72-7). By breathing in inverted and semi-inverted positions, the pressure of the diaphragm is taken off the lower lungs and upper abdominal organs, and this helps gently to massage and tone them. Above all, flushing the brain with an extra supply of blood for a few short moments has a calming influence on the mind and is therefore very useful for stress relief.

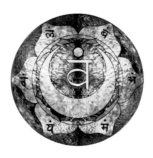

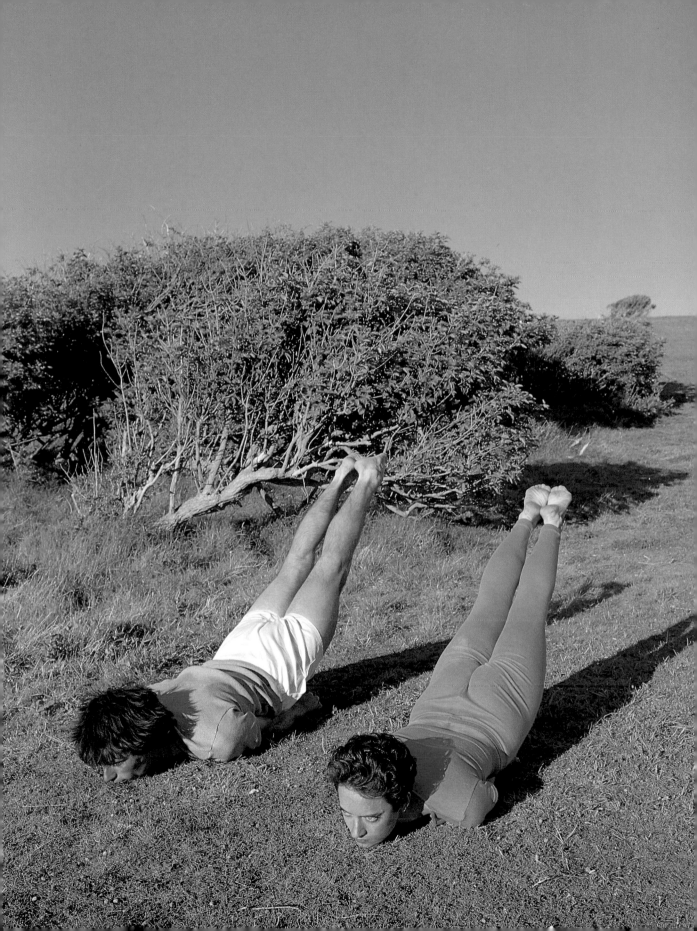

BOWING-DOWN POSES

Bowing-Down postures help to stretch the spine and the back muscles, regenerating the spinal nerves and releasing tension. Breathing with the abdomen pressed against the thighs enables the movement of the diaphragm gently to massage the internal organs.

    Practise all of these postures with your eyes closed. This will help you to maintain inner calm.

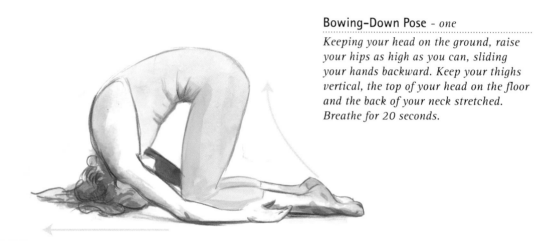

Bowing-Down Pose - *one*

Keeping your head on the ground, raise your hips as high as you can, sliding your hands backward. Keep your thighs vertical, the top of your head on the floor and the back of your neck stretched. Breathe for 20 seconds.

USEFUL TIP

If you are over thirty years of age you should practise weightbearing exercises such as the Half-Headstand regularly to help counteract the gradual decline in your bone density.

Bowing-Down Pose - *two*

Inhale. Exhaling, lower your buttocks on to your heels. Relax your neck, with your forehead on the ground. Breathe normally. Stretch your arms forward, with your palms on the floor. Breathe for 10 seconds. Repeat twice. Sit up, inhaling, and exhale.

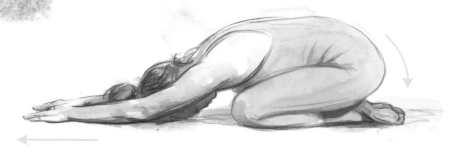

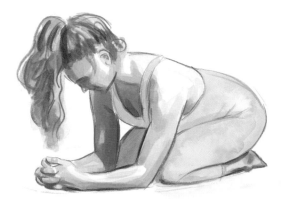

The Half-Headstand - *one*

Kneel down with your legs together, resting on your heels. Place your elbows on the ground in front of your knees. The distance between them should be the length of your forearm. Interlink your fingers, to form a triangle.

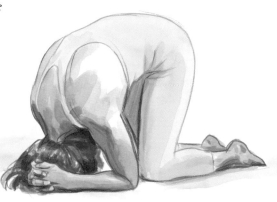

The Half-Headstand - *two*

Place the front part of the crown of your head on the ground. Rest the back of your head against your palms.

THE HALF-HEADSTAND

The Half-Headstand is so called because it is often used to prepare the body for the Headstand, although it is a posture in its own right. In both these postures most of the body's weight is taken on the forearms and shoulders, and not on the head. The Half-Headstand is a valuable posture because it strengthens the arms and shoulder muscles; areas of the body which are often quite under-developed and weak. It is also very beneficial because it requires weightbearing on the upper limbs. This mechanically stresses the arm bones, and weightbearing stress is an important factor in the maintenance of the mineral content of the bones.

After practising the inverted postures, lie down on your front with your head to one side, your legs stretched out behind you, your big toes touching and your heels turned outward, and your arms by your sides. Relax for a minute or two.

The Half-Headstand - *three*

Keeping your forearms, hands and head firmly on the floor, raise your hips until your knees are straight. Breathe for 10 seconds. Pressing your toes and forearms into the ground, lift your hips further up. Let your forearms support your body weight and put very little weight on your head. Walk your toes toward your head so that your back is as straight as possible. Breathe for 20 seconds.

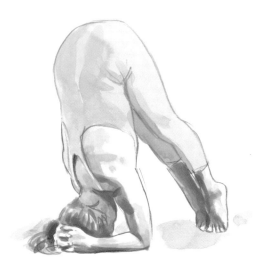

The Half-Headstand - *four*

Inhale, hold your breath, lower your knees to the floor, and your buttocks on to your heels, exhaling, while placing your hands separately on the ground by the side of your head, and sliding the palms forward. Move your arms backward as in the Child Pose (see p.93). Breathe normally.

The Dog Pose – Swanasana

Repeat steps one, two and three. Keeping your head and feet on the ground, place your hands on the floor by the side of your head. Pressing them into the ground, lift your head up and straighten your elbows. Support your body weight with your feet. Let your head hang down between your arms. Relax your neck. Breathe for 20 seconds. Inhale, hold your breath and exhaling, lower your knees and buttocks, as in step four. Breathe for 10 seconds and sit up.

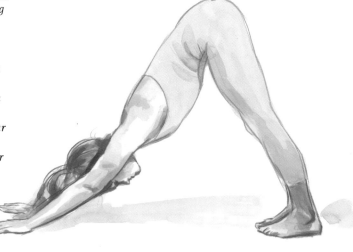

The Child Pose - *one*

Sit on your heels. Place your hands on them. Bend backward, with your head back, inhaling.

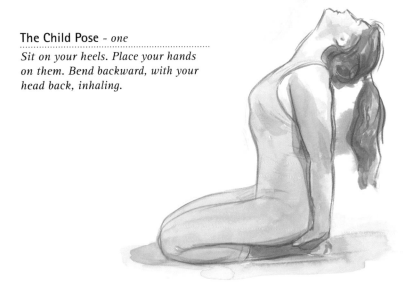

The Child Pose - *two*

Bend forward slowly, exhaling. Place your forehead on the ground close to your knees, letting go of your heels. Place the backs of your hands on the floor. Relax your neck and shoulders. Breathe for 10 seconds. Feel peaceful and at rest.

THE CHILD POSE

The Child Pose is a good posture to rest in for a minute or two after doing a sequence of basic asanas. It gives a powerful forward stretch to the spine of 110°, relaxing the spinal ligaments and stretching the back muscles. It helps to alleviate the compression of the lower invertebral discs, which occurs when we are standing. In addition breathing with the abdomen resting on the thighs allows the diaphragm to gently stimulate the internal organs with a light massage. It also improves the circulation in the face which is beneficial for the eyes, the ears and the facial muscles.

COBRA POSE – BHUJANGASANA

The Cobra Pose is one of the most important *asanas*. The arching of the spine improves its flexibility, and rejuvenates the spinal nerves. The state of the spine influences our general health, both physical and mental, because the spinal cord channels the nerve impulses to and from the brain all over the body.

This posture puts gentle pressure on the abdomen and massages the internal organs. It is a very useful pose for alleviating menstrual disorders and ovarian and uterine problems.

The curving of the back helps to massage the adrenal glands. It is important to keep the adrenal glands in good working order as they help to control our response to stress, and our metabolism.

USEFUL TIP
Come into the posture in three stages.
Be careful not to hunch your shoulders and to keep your face relaxed.

Cobra Pose - *one*

Place your palms by the side of your chest, the tips of your fingers in line with your shoulders, so that your elbows are close to your sides. Place your forehead on the ground and keep your toes facing backward.

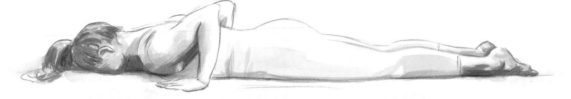

Cobra Pose - *two*

First stretch your neck by pressing your chin into your chest. Move your head backward, inhaling, counting up to three, your palms lightly resting on the floor. Shoulders relaxed. Hold your breath.

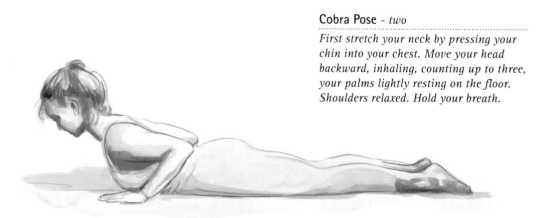

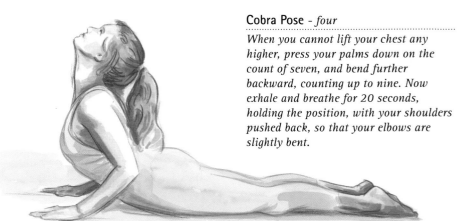

Cobra Pose - *three*

Raise your chest, keeping your head back and palms slightly raised. Counting from four to six, press your lower abdomen and pelvis into the ground.

Cobra Pose - *four*

When you cannot lift your chest any higher, press your palms down on the count of seven, and bend further backward, counting up to nine. Now exhale and breathe for 20 seconds, holding the position, with your shoulders pushed back, so that your elbows are slightly bent.

Cobra Pose - *five*

Inhale deeply and hold your breath. Keeping your head back, lower your chest, counting up to three. On the count of four, raise your palms slightly. Exhale slowly, lowering your chest but keeping your head back. Count from five to seven, resting your chin and palms on the ground. On the count of eight and nine, move your head forward, letting your forehead touch the floor. Breathe for 10 seconds. Repeat once and rest.

MOON POSE – SHASHANKASANA

The Locust should not be done immediately after the Cobra, since it is another backward stretch. Instead practise a counterpose in-between, to relieve tension in the lower back. You can do this in the Moon Pose from the lying-down position.

You have already done part of the Moon Pose in the last part of the Bowing-Down Pose (see p.90). The backward and forward movements of the Moon Pose exercise the spine and muscles of the torso. By holding this posture for several breaths, you gain the same benefits as in the Child Pose (see p.93).

Moon Pose - *one*

Having rested for a while after the Cobra Pose, place your palms on the ground by the side of your head.

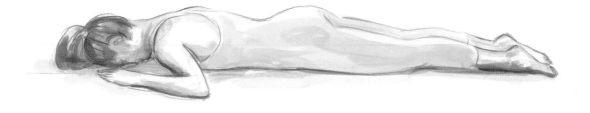

Moon Pose - *two*

Inhale and hold your breath. Pressing your palms and knees into the floor, lift and push your hips backward.

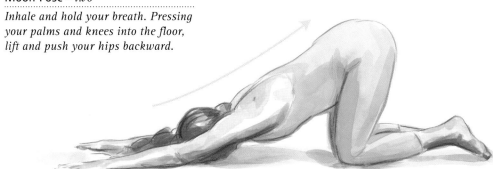

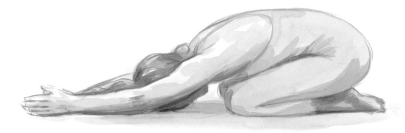

Moon Pose - *three*

Exhaling, slide your hands back, until your buttocks are resting on your heels. Now, stretching your arms out in front, bring your palms together, with your thumbs crossed. Breathe for 20 seconds.

Moon Pose - *four*

Slide your folded palms toward your head until your wrists touch your head. Breathe for 10 seconds.

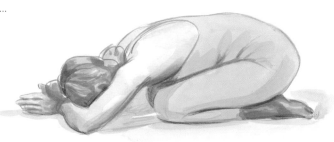

Moon Pose - *five*

Move your arms back. Join your palms above your hips, your fingers pointing backward. Breathe for 10 seconds. Stretch your arms forward and place your palms on the ground. Inhale and hold your breath. Pressing your palms into the ground, push your forehead forward, exhaling, until your chest and abdomen are flat on the floor. Lower your arms by your sides and rest for a minute.

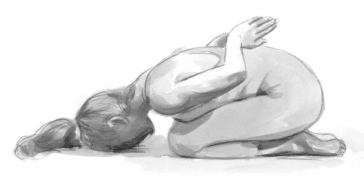

LOCUST–SALABHASANA

The Locust complements the Cobra Pose (see pp.94-5), and completes the Backward Bend (see p.60). This posture strengthens the shoulder, buttock, back and leg muscles, and maintains flexibility of the spine. As in the Cobra, it massages the abdominal organs, regulating the digestion, and in addition has an even stronger effect on the pelvic area.

Start with the Half-Locust and then move on to the full Locust. At first you will find it difficult to raise your legs very far off the floor. However with regular practice and perseverance you will gradually develop more muscular strength and be able to raise them higher.

CAUTION
Having raised both legs off the floor, if you find it too difficult to move them apart, avoid this. If, however, you can do this, it will help to massage the pelvis.

Half-Locust - *one*

Lie down on your stomach, chin on the ground, arms by your sides, legs straight. Clench your fists and bring them together under your groin, the back of your hands on the floor. Hold your fists in whatever position gives you the most leverage. The idea is to raise your legs, pressing your fists into the floor.

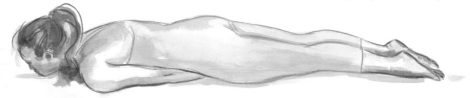

Half-Locust - *two*

Inhale deeply, hold your breath and raise your left leg as high as you can, without bending your knees, pressing your fists and shoulders into the ground. Do not put pressure on your right leg, raise your hip off the floor, or rotate the leg outward. Keep holding your breath for five seconds. Then lower your leg, exhaling. Take a couple of breaths. Do the same on the right side. Repeat once on each side.

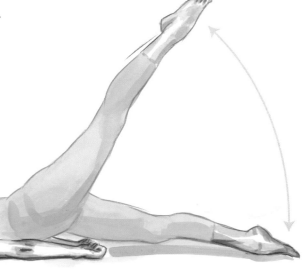

Locust - *one*

Lie down in the same starting position as for the Half-Locust, step one.

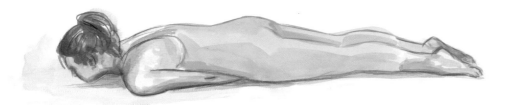

Locust - *two*

After taking a few normal breaths, inhale deeply, hold your breath, and raise both legs in the same way. Hold, breathing for five seconds. Then lower your legs, exhaling. Repeat once and breathe normally.

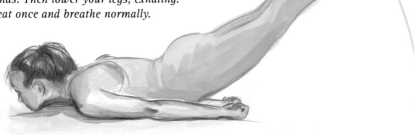

Locust - *three*

Inhale and hold your breath. Keeping your arms and hands stretched out behind you flat on the floor, raise both legs. Then move them apart as much as you can, exhaling. Bring them together in the raised position, inhaling. Repeat once. Lower your legs, exhaling.

Place your arms by your sides, with the palms facing up, and rest with your head to one side for a minute or two.

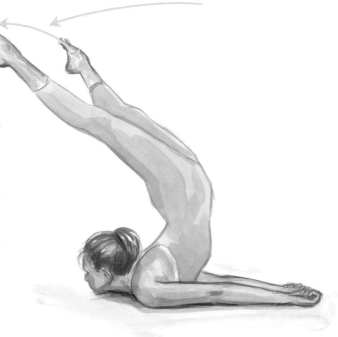

CAT POSE – VYAGHRASANA

Before doing the Bow Pose (see pp.102-3), you should do a counterpose such as the Cat Pose. This exercises the spine and is helpful for stress relief. The upward and downward movement of the torso, and stretching and flexing of the legs, increases the flexibility of the spine and strengthens the legs.

   In the Cat Pose the back is stretched and arched in a forward, then backward direction. This stretches the back muscles. It also moves the small facet joints between the backs of the vertebrae, helping to maintain full mobility of the spine.

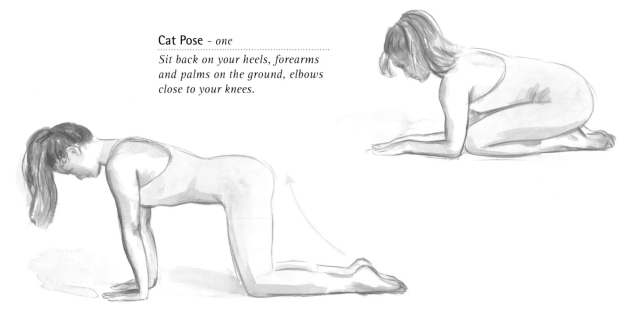

Cat Pose - *one*

Sit back on your heels, forearms and palms on the ground, elbows close to your knees.

Cat Pose - *two*

Raise your hips and shoulders, straightening your arms. Breathe normally. Inhale.

Cat Pose - *three*

Then, arching your back as high as you can, exhale and lower your head between your arms. Breathe normally.

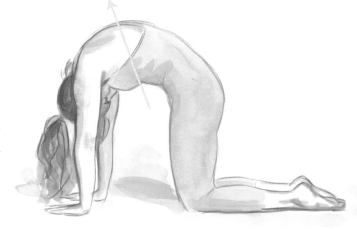

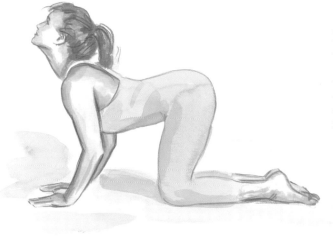

Cat Pose - *four*

Inhaling, dip your chest down, bending the elbows slightly, and lift your head up. Hold your breath for five seconds. Exhaling, lift your back up as before (see step three), and repeat twice. Sit back on your heels and breathe normally.

Cat Pose - *five*

Assume the position in step two, and take several breaths. Inhaling, stretch the left leg backward and as high up as you can, lifting your head up and dipping your chest a little, bending your elbows slightly. Hold your breath for five seconds.

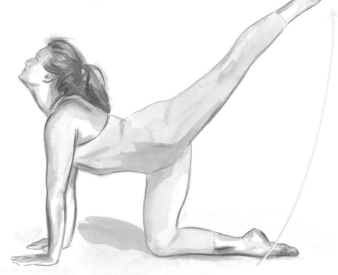

Cat Pose - *six*

Exhaling, bend your left knee forward, straightening your arms and arching your back, bending your forehead on to your knee. Take a normal breath. Repeat once. Lower your knee and return to the position in step two. Take a normal breath again. Repeat twice with the right leg. Lower the knee, sit back on your heels, and breathe normally.

BOW POSE – DHANURASANA

The Bow Pose combines the effect of both the Cobra (see pp.94-5), and the Locust (see pp.98-9). In this posture, even greater pressure is placed on the abdominal organs, and the whole of the spine is arched backward, from the neck to the lower back. This helps to release tension in the spine and solar plexus, and to counteract mental and physical sluggishness.

By massaging the pancreas, the Bow Pose helps to balance and regulate the secretion of glycogen and insulin. It also improves the working of the kidneys, which flush and purify the blood better. The whole length of the alimentary canal is toned, and any sluggishness of the liver and large and small intestines is remedied. It also stimulates the stomach glands, helping digestion, and improves the function of the adrenals and thyroid glands, reducing hyperactivity and countering lethargy.

USEFUL TIPS
Before doing the full Bow, prepare yourself by practising the Half-Bow stretches on either side.
Following the Bow, relax in the Child Pose (see p.93) for a short while.
It is easier to do this posture with your knees apart. If you are fairly supple you can practise with them together.

Half-Bow - *one*

Lie on your stomach, your forehead on the ground. Stretch your right arm forward. Hold your right foot, if possible at the ankle, with your left hand. Breathe for five seconds.

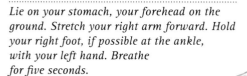

Half-Bow - *two*

Inhaling, arch backward, lifting your right knee off the ground, tilt your head back and right arm up. Keep your left leg flat on the floor. Hold and breathe for five seconds. Exhaling, lower your right knee, chest, forehead and right arm to the ground. Breathe normally, and repeat the stretch. Repeat twice on the other side. Rest with your head to one side.

Bow Pose - *one*

Lie on your stomach, with your forehead on the ground, arms by your sides, and your legs stretched out behind you.

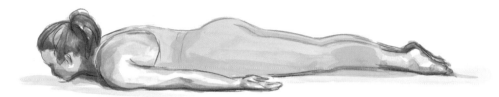

Bow Pose - *two*

Clasp hold of your feet or ankles, keeping your big toes close together. Take a few normal breaths.

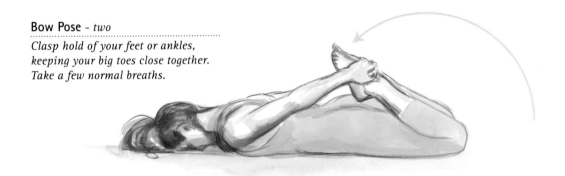

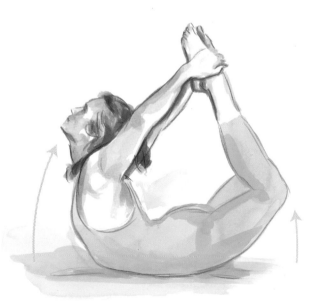

Bow Pose - *three*

Pull your feet up, arching back, tilting your head back, inhaling. Let the weight of your body rest on the lower abdomen, pelvis and upper thighs. Hold your breath for five seconds. Exhaling, lower your knees, chest and forehead to the ground. Breathe for 10 seconds. Repeat once.

Once in the Bow Pose you can rock foward, exhaling and backward, inhaling, several times, and sideways from left to right. This will give your internal organs a strong massage.

SIMPLE–SPINAL TWIST – MERU-VAKRASANA

Although this posture does not belong to the Cobra series
(see pp.94-105), you can conclude the sequence by doing this
simple form of spinal twist to balance the stretches. It completes
the exercise of the spinal column, and the organs inside the thorax.

   You can practise this as preparation for a more complex form
of the spinal twist, *Ardha-Matsyendrasana*, or the Half-Spinal
Twist (see p.105).

> **PRANAYAMA & MEDITATION**
> To complete this routine
> relax for five minutes in the
> Corpse Pose (see p.52), and
> follow with the breathing
> exercises on pp.53-5, and
> then the 15 minute
> meditation (see p.87).

Simple–Spinal Twist - *one*

*Sit with your legs straight out in front of
you. Place your left foot across your
right knee on the ground. Cradle your
left knee in the crook of your right
elbow, with your palm on your left
thigh. Hold your left hip up. Put your
left arm behind your back, keeping the
back of your hand on the right side of
your waist. Twist your head to the left
and slightly up. Push your left shoulder
back. Breathe for 20 seconds.*

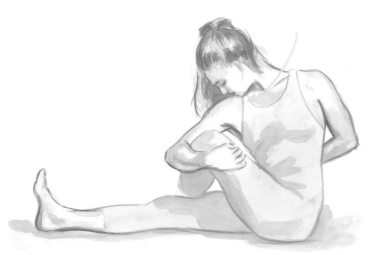

Simple–Spinal Twist - *two*

*Inhale and hold your breath. Exhaling,
bend your head down, place your chin on
your chest, and roll your chin to the right
until your nose touches your right arm.
Do not lift your head. Push your left
shoulder forward. Breathe for 10
seconds. Inhaling, roll your chin in the
same way to the left. Push back your left
shoulder. Hold your breath for 5 seconds
and exhale. Repeat once. Repeat steps
one and two on the other side. Relax.*

HALF-SPINAL TWIST

The Half-Spinal Twist or *Ardha-Matsyendrasana* is named after the great yogic sage, Matsyendra, one of the early teachers of *Hatha* yoga. This *asana* gives a sideways stretch to the spine, back muscles and hips. It massages the abdominal muscles, alleviating digestive disorders. It also tones the spinal nerves and ligaments, and the sympathetic nervous system. It is a useful pose to practise for relieving muscular tension in the back and hips.

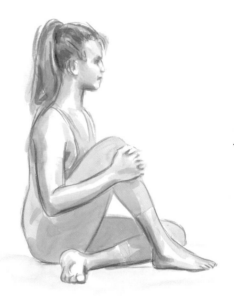

Half-Spinal Twist - *one*

Sit on your heels, keeping your back straight. With your knees bent, lower your hips to the floor so that you are sitting to the left of your feet. Raise your right knee and place the right foot flat on the floor. Let your left leg turn on its side, with the left foot below the right leg.

Half-Spinal Twist - *two*

Place your right foot across your left knee and your left foot under your right hip. Hold your right leg at the ankle, if possible with your left hand. Place your right forearm across your lower back, keeping the back of your hand on the left of your waist. Twist to the right, turning your head to the right. Hold, breathing freely for 10 seconds. Release your arms, inhaling. Face forward and lower your arms, exhaling. Stretch your legs out in front of you. Repeat on the opposite side.

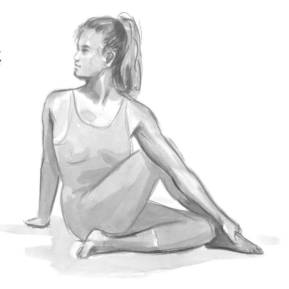

CHAPTER SEVEN

Weeks nine and ten

In the ninth week, you can replace the lumbar bends and stretches from weeks three and four (see pp.60-9), with the twelve postures of *Surya-Namaskara*, or the Sun Salutation (see pp.108-9). This is an all-round exercise which involves and invigorates the whole body. These postures used to be practised a long time ago, facing the rising sun, each with the intonation of a *mantra*. Ideally you would practise these in the sun (although not in its direct heat), preferably outside, or in a sunny room, for a truly invigorating result. When there is no sun it helps to imagine its presence.

Although the Sun Salutation is not considered to be part of the traditional practice of *asanas* in *Hatha yoga*, it does include many of the traditional postures. The movements stretch and energise the whole body, loosen up the joints and massage the internal organs and glands. They also improve the blood circulation and breathing. Afterwards, your body and mind will be fully relaxed.

Throughout the sequence you should breathe in rhythm with your movements. Do not forget to inhale and exhale in each of the postures. To gain maximum benefit, you should practise this sequence slowly, not dynamically. Do not swing from one posture to another, but pause for seven seconds between each stage.

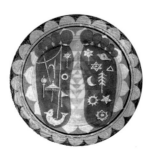

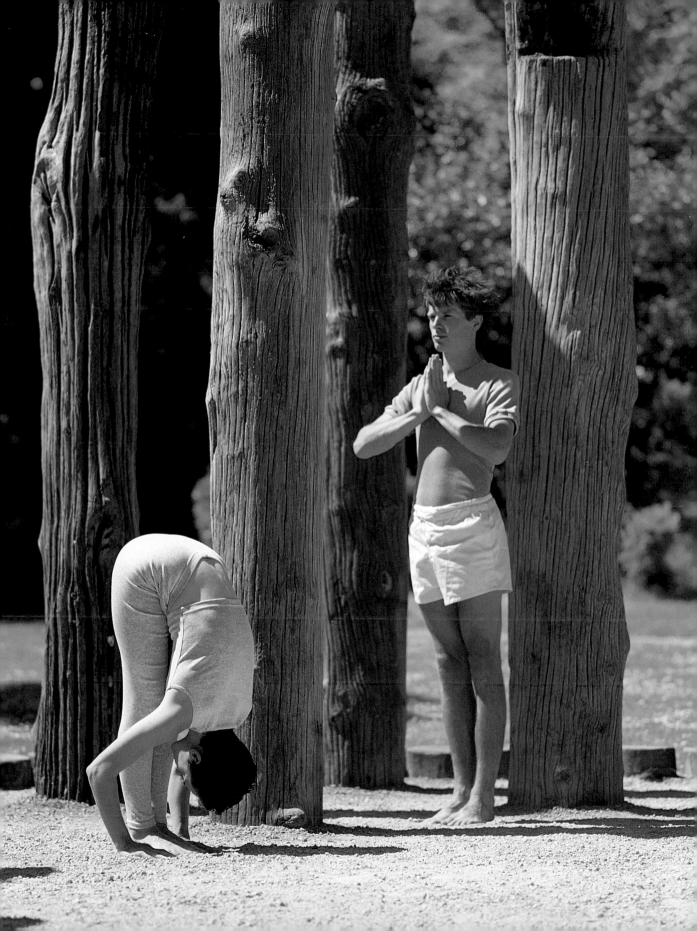

SUN SALUTATION

Preparation for the pose

Stand up straight, with your feet together, arms loose by your sides. Relax your shoulders and legs. Place your right forearm on your left shoulder and your left forearm on your lower back.

Twist to the left, turning your head to the left, giving a gentle squeeze to the back. Twist to the right and do the same. Repeat once more on each side. Face forward, relax your shoulders and legs.

Now you are ready for the Sun Salutation.

Sun Salutation - *one*

Stand up straight, with your feet touching and your palms together on your chest.
Inhale.

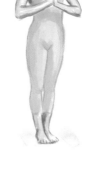

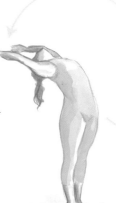

Sun Salutation - *two*

Exhaling, bend forward. Link your right thumb over your left. Stretch your arms forward and raise them up, inhaling, arch back, and breathe for seven seconds.

USEFUL TIP

In the first week, do only two rounds. Then lie down and rest in the Corpse Pose (see p.52) for two to three minutes.

In the second week, while doing the two rounds, you can add *Agnisara* (see p.85), in steps three, eight and ten, to increase the effect on the abdominal organs.

Sun Salutation - *three*

Stretch up, inhaling, and bend forward exhaling, bringing your head to your knees and lining your finger tips up with your toes. Take a few deep breaths.

Sun Salutation - *four*

Inhale, stretch your left leg back, keeping your left toes tucked under and look up.

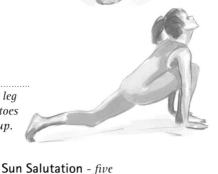

Sun Salutation - *five*

Inhaling, stretch both legs back, keeping your body in a straight line. Rest your weight on your hands and toes. Take a few breaths.

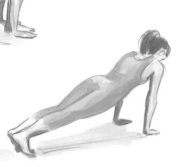

Sun Salutation - *twelve*

Stretch up, inhaling, and lower your arms, exhaling. Bring your palms together. Loosen up as in the preparation for the pose (see p.108).
Repeat, starting on the right side.

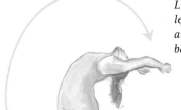

Sun Salutation - *eleven*

Linking the right thumb over the left, stretch your arms forward and inhaling, rise up and stretch back. Take a few breaths.

Sun Salutation - *ten*

Inhale, and exhaling, bring your legs forward. Keeping your knees straight, bring your head to your knees, finger tips lined up with your toes. Take a few breaths.

Sun Salutation - *nine*

Inhale, bring your left foot forward between your hands, your right toes tucked under. Look up. Take a few breaths.

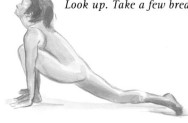

Sun Salutation - *eight*

Inhale, and exhaling, come up into the Dog Pose. Bring your heels down to the floor and move your hips up. Take a few breaths.

Sun Salutation - *six*

Inhale, place your chest and knees on the floor, exhaling. Keep your hips slightly raised and your toes tucked under. Take a few breaths.

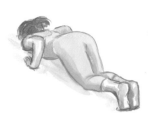

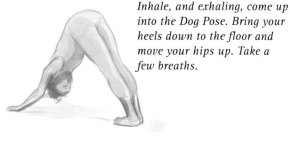

Sun Salutation - *seven*

Inhaling, press down with your hands, raise your head and chest, keeping your hips on the floor, elbows bent, and your feet stretched back. Shoulders pulled back. Take a few breaths.

CLEANSING BREATH - KAPALABHATI

In the tenth week, after doing *Nadi-Sodhana pranayama* (see pp.53-4), followed by *Ujjayi* (see p.55), you can replace *Shitali* and *Shitakari* (see p.86) by *Kapalabhati*. *Kapala* means forehead or skull, and *bhati* means cleansing. In this exercise your lungs work like bellows, pumping air forcefully in and out. This *pranayama* is particularly useful for stress relief because it cleanses the system, calms the mind and generates *prana* throughout the body. As the abdomen is sharply and rapidly contracted, lifting up the diaphragm and then relaxed, this exercises and clears the lower lungs. It also improves their elasticity and increases your breathing capacity. The forceful movement of the abdomen massages the internal organs.

By emptying the stale air from your lungs, you make way for a fresh intake of oxygen-rich air which helps to purify the blood, to strengthen the circulation and to cleanse the entire respiratory system. In this way, you clear the mind, improve concentration and reach a state of inner calm.

CAUTION
If you feel giddy, stop and breathe normally for a while, and then resume the practice.
Do not do this *pranayama* if you are pregnant or suffering from high blood pressure.

Cleansing Breath - *one*

Sit in a comfortable position, with your shoulders and back straight. Breathe deeply and slowly twice, to relax your lungs.

Cleansing Breath - *three*

After sharply exhaling for the last time, inhale deeply and exhale slowly and fully. Do so twice more. Then inhale slowly, holding your breath, press your chin against your chest, keeping your shoulders straight (Jalandhara-Bandha) and contract the rectal muscles (Mula-Bandha). Hold your breath in this position for 30 seconds. Concentrate on the beating of your heart.

Lift up your head and relax your rectal muscles, exhaling. Breathe normally. Do one more round.

Lie down and relax in the Corpse Pose (see p.52) for five minutes, if you wish to complete the session with meditation. Otherwise, relax for 10 minutes and meditate later at a convenient time.

By breathing deeply you relax the lungs and by putting on the bandhas *(muscular locks or contractions), you help to absorb the* prana *generated during rapid breathing.*

Cleansing Breath - *two*

Inhale normally, letting your abdomen expand, then forcefully exhale, sharply contracting it. Immediately inhale gently, relaxing your abdomen, and let your lungs fill with air.

Begin by inhaling and exhaling 50 times in 30 seconds. In the final two weeks, aim to increase your speed to 60 breaths in 30 seconds.

USEFUL TIPS
Throughout this exercise, keep your eyes closed, concentrating on your sinuses.
While breathing rapidly, do not contract the facial muscles.

MEDITATION

Begin by practising the same meditation as in the previous days (see p.87). Then, after a minute of relaxation, keeping your eyes closed and breathing normally, concentrate on the in- and out-flow of the *prana*, the coolness inside your head and the warmth within your lower nostrils. Do this for a minute.

Now move on to the next stage, which you should do for at least five minutes.

Repeat to yourself, inhaling and feeling the coolness, "Peace is my real nature", and exhaling and experiencing the warmth, "not conflict". Try to believe in what you are saying. Then, letting your mind gently float with the breath, be aware of the breath, the coolness absorbing and making grooves of peace in the subconscious, and the warmth smoothing and easing any thoughts or feelings of conflict, stress and inner tension.

You may choose phrases to suit your specific need, depending on the cause of your stress.

Select a few affirmations for each session and use them for as long as you need to. From time to time, alter the affirmations to suit your mood.

Detach your mind, and relax for two minutes, breathing normally and feeling peaceful and restful, before getting up.

"Detachment is my real nature", inhaling,
"not attachment", exhaling.
"Freedom is my real nature", "not bondage".
"Humility is my real nature", "not self-importance".
"Patience is my real nature", "not impatience".
"Tolerance is my real nature", "not intolerance".
"Love is my real nature", "not resentment", (or "hate").
"Truth is my real nature", "not dishonesty".
"Caring is my real nature", "not selfishness".

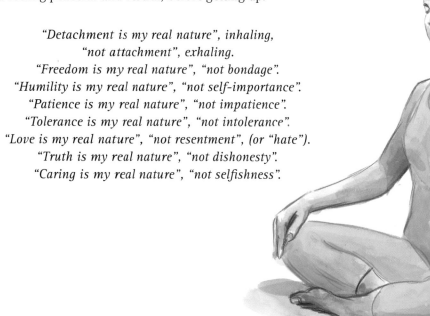

CHAPTER EIGHT

Weeks eleven and twelve

Follow the same routine as in weeks nine and ten, but increase your practice of the Sun Salutation, from two to four rounds.

Repeat *Kapalabhati*, the breathing exercise from weeks nine and ten (see p.110), then follow with a very simple form of *Yoga Nidra*, a deep and longer relaxation (see pp.114-17). *Yoga Nidra* means yogic sleep, but is actually a wakeful state of deep introversion. In the initial stages, it involves relaxing the body, part by part, and harmonising the mind. It is an inner awareness, a movement of consciousness, rather than a deliberate auto-suggestion. You cannot relax by trying to relax, but by feeling relaxed, for "trying" means making an effort.

Having relaxed your body and calmed your mind, you can plant a few intentions, *sankalpas*, in your subconscious, before detaching your mind and experiencing the final stage of deep relaxation. Choose suggestions which match your needs, like the affirmations from the meditation in the previous weeks.

Before beginning you should do some exercises to warm up your whole body. If you are short of time, you can start with the nine stretches from weeks one and two, involving the shoulder and neck muscles (see pp.40-7) and then do two rounds of the Sun Salutation (see pp.108-9). Following this, relax in *Yoga Nidra* for twenty minutes.

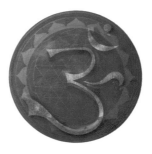

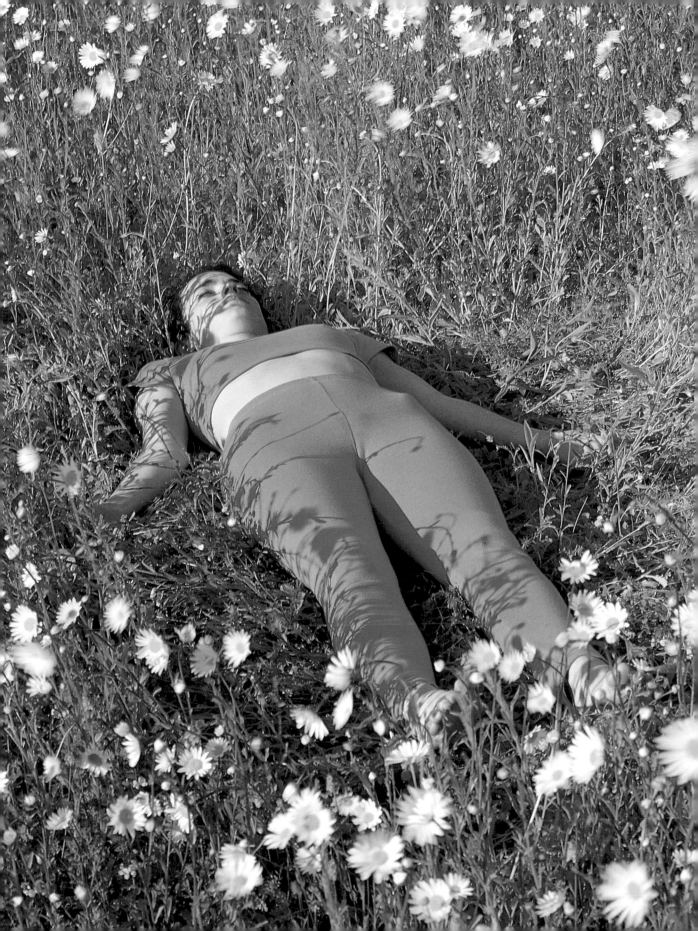

DEEP RELAXATION – YOGA NIDRA

Before starting, tape the *Yoga Nidra* sequence either yourself or have it recorded by someone whose voice you like. If you play the tape at low volume it will help to guide you through the practice, and allow you to benefit fully from the relaxation. Before going into the full pose, prepare yourself by relaxing each part of your body in turn. Lie down in the Corpse Pose (see p.52). Detach your mind and close your eyes, breathe normally. Do not "try" to do anything, not even to relax. After a minute, loosen up your body, part by part, with slight movements.

Yoga Nidra - *before you start*

Relax your toes. Flex your ankles. Loosen up your legs, without bending your knees. Roll your hips from left to right, and lower them down. Lift them up and down, gently. Relax the lower part of your body.

Move your fingers. Flex your wrists. Relax your arms and shoulders. Keeping your head and hips on the ground, lift your chest gently up and down. Roll your head from left to right. Keep your head straight. Relax the upper part of your body. Detach your mind, and lie peacefully for a minute.

Now you can practise "the Rotation of Awareness". As you move your mind from one part of the body to another, keep your body still.

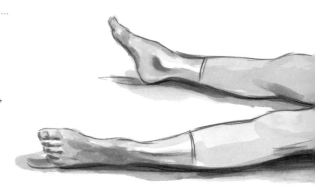

Yoga Nidra - *one*

Be aware of your left toes, one by one, from the little to the big toe, the sole of the foot, the heel, the ankle, the top of the foot and back again to the toes. Move your mind from your left ankle up your leg to the knee, becoming aware of the calf muscles, your shin bone, your knee joint, then downward, feeling the relaxation and regeneration of each part. Imagine the flow of prana, or a gentle current, along the leg, upward as you inhale and downward as you exhale. Repeat a few times. Move your mind up your thigh, from your knee to your pelvis, and down again. Be aware of the muscles, bones, ligaments and joints, as you inhale and exhale freely.

Repeat along the right leg.

USEFUL TIPS

Do not focus your mind on your breath, but on the parts of your body.

See your body as an object and your mind as an instrument of your inner spirit directing the flow of *prana* into your body. With each part of the body imagine the flow of *prana* relaxing and revitalising the whole part, as you inhale and exhale freely.

Keep the room well ventilated, and the temperature at 22°C (72°F).

Cover yourself with a blanket.

Yoga Nidra - *six*

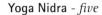

*Be aware of your throat and neck, the
back of your head, your jaws, your
cheeks, your chin, your lips and nose.
The inside of your mouth and nose, your
left eye-lid and inside of the eye, the
same with the right eye, your left and
right eyebrow, your forehead. Relax it.
Move to your left and right temple, your
left ear and inside it, the same with the
right ear, then the top of your head. Feel
the coolness of your breath inside your
head, as you inhale. Detach your mind,
and lie peacefully for about five minutes.*

Yoga Nidra - *five*

*Be aware of the fingers of your left hand,
from the little finger to the thumb, the
palms, the back of your hand and wrist.
Move upward along your forearm, from
the wrist to the elbow, and downward.
Repeat with your upper arm. Do the
same with the right arm.*

Yoga Nidra - *four*

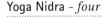

*Be aware of the movement of your
chest, feeling the relaxation and
regeneration of the muscles.*

*Place your awareness in your left
lung, then the right lung, the
bronchial tubes connecting the
trachea, up and down it, and along
the oesophagus. Then feel your heartbeat. Move your awareness from the
left kidney to the right.*

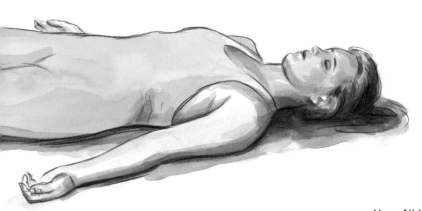

Yoga Nidra - *two*

*Be aware of the rise and full of your
abdomen, as you inhale and exhale. Feel
the muscles relaxing and being
regenerated.*

*Move your mind to your abdominal
organs. Dwell on each for a few seconds:
the colon, the bladder, the sexual organs,
the intestines, the spleen to the lower
left, and the liver to the upper right, the
pancreas, the stomach.*

Yoga Nidra - *three*

*Be aware of your buttocks, your lower
and upper back. Move your mind along
the spine upward and downward, from
the coccyx to the cervical vertebrae,
feeling the regeneration of the discs,
joints and the spinal cord. Synchronise
the movement with your breath, inhaling
with the upward breath and exhaling
with the downward.*

MEDITATIVE VISUALISATIONS

There are many different techniques you can use in *Yoga Nidra*. One of the most effective is to concentrate on the flow of the breath. You can use the inward and outward flow of the breath to develop an awareness of an inner peace. With the in-breath you can imagine the peacefulness flowing into your being and with the outward breath, the inner tension flowing out. Gradually, once you have mastered this awareness, you can plant a few intentions in your subconscious, using words such as "peace" and "freedom".

Visualising images is more of a challenge. Start with very simple images such as a clear blue sky, and slowly progress to more complex images such as a meadow and surrounding woods.

Visualise a clear
blue sky, a symbol of
the infinite spirit, of love
and goodness, enveloping you.
Then an open field, with its light-
green grass. It is your subconscious.
In the distance, dark-green woods
surround it. They are your unconscious.
Imagine a gentle breeze, the universal energy,
smoothing out the grass, all inner conflicts,
and penetrating into the woods, ventilating the
deep recesses of the unconscious, purifying and
sublimating its nature.

Relax your mind, and remain detached for a while.

Now plant into your subconscious three intentions, which
you can choose to suit you, such as:

I should take things calmly and practise detachment.

I should restrain impulsive reaction and hold my tongue.

I should practise tolerance and patience.

Detach your
mind after several
minutes of deep relaxation.
Now be aware of your body.
Slowly turn on one side and curl
up in the foetal position, and rest
for a few minutes. Then get up.
There are other forms of visualisation.
You can try one of the following:

Imagine a deep-blue sea, with gently rolling
waves. You are one of the waves. Be aware of it
slowly rising and falling, along with the rhythm
of your breath. The light-blue sky above is the
infinite spirit, of love and goodness, enveloping all
the waves. There is no division, no judgement, no
aggression. Profound peace flows like a gentle breeze,
slowly swaying the cradle of life.

FINALLY

Throughout your yoga practice keep the following basic rules in mind:
Think positively and treat others with respect.

....

Exercise self-discipline in your eating, sleeping and work habits.

....

Exercise regularly - try to do the equivalent of three miles brisk walking or one
hour of yoga postures and fifteen minutes of breathing exercises each day.

....

Focus on improving your breathing, and your posture.
Be conscious of keeping your torso straight.

....

Learn to relax, both physically and mentally.

....

Light and shadow are a part of life. We all possess the capacity to develop excellent
qualities, and there are many positive aspects of life from which we can learn. The
essence of yoga is to learn to appreciate the happier moments in life and to take in
our stride the unhappier ones without rancour. In the spirit of St Francis of Assisi, we
should have "the courage to change what can be changed and the serenity to accept
what cannot be, and the wisdom to know what can be changed and what cannot be".

PART THREE

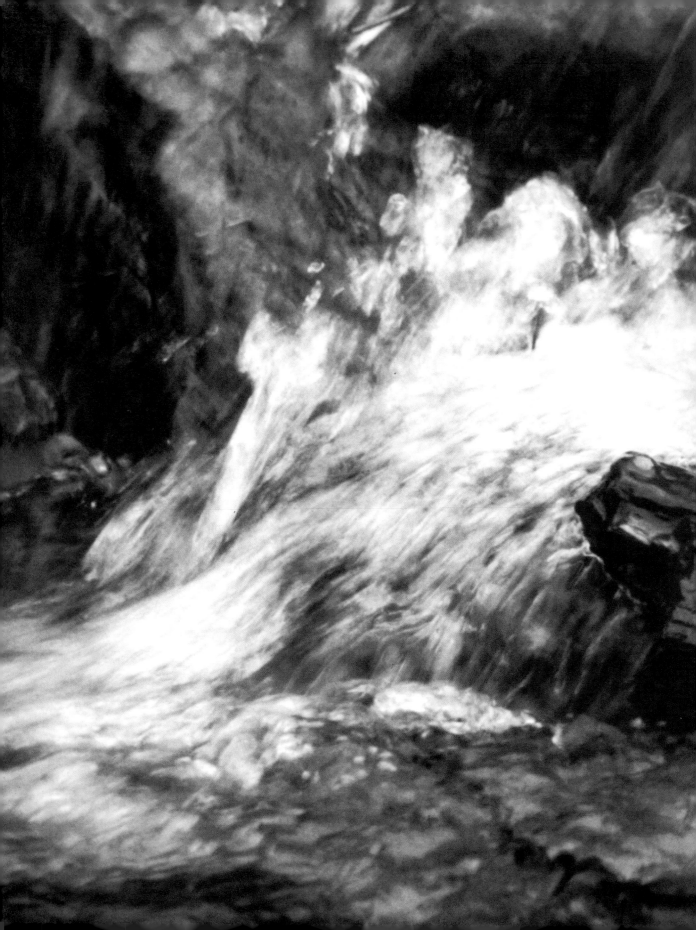

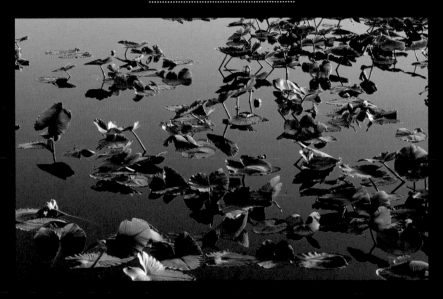

Overcoming Stress–Related Ailments

"Lower your level of expectation, practise detachment, exercise regularly, and be balanced in your eating and sleeping habits."

USING YOGA TO RESTORE HEALTH

At some stage in our lives we will all experience some degree of ill-health. When stress exceeds normal levels it may weaken the immune system and make the body more susceptible to infection. Moreover, stress may, in some cases, contribute to the development of disorders such as hypertension, heart disease, peptic ulcers, digestive problems and many other ailments. Illness may in addition be the result of an imbalance in our energy body when the flow of *prana* becomes blocked. Yoga assists in restoring equilibrium to the body and mind so that good health can flourish. It is particularly effective at dealing with stress-related disorders, because it works at both a physical and mental level. The *asanas* work on the physical body, and the breathing exercises, and meditation practices, help to control and calm the mind.

Part Three looks at twelve commonplace stress-related ailments, and illustrates how to use specific *asanas*, breathing exercises and meditation practices selected from the Three-Month Programme (see pp.35-117) to alleviate and overcome these disorders. Cardio-vascular disorders including heart disease and hypertension, digestive ailments, diabetes, asthma, arthritis and headaches, are all covered. Several conditions which are largely pyschological in origin, such as anxiety, panic attacks, insomnia, depression and addiction are also dealt with.

Advice is given on the benefits of yoga for the elderly and pregnant women. Yoga is an ideal form of exercise for people in later life because it helps to maintain suppleness in the limbs and to strengthen the muscles, making one less susceptible to illnesses such as arthritis and rheumatism. It can also be very beneficial in pregnancy, both in alleviating symptoms such as varicose veins and nausea, and in preparing for the birth.

Always bear in mind that although yoga can bring you great benefits, it is not meant as a substitute for conventional medical care. Be sure to consult your doctor and follow any treatment prescribed, in addition to using yoga therapy, and if you are suffering from a serious condition, you should practise yoga with the help of a qualified yoga therapist.

However, anyone with only minor ailments, such as slightly raised blood pressure, tension headaches, backache due to muscular strain and chronic tension, can safely practise any of the exercises from the Three-Month Programme to prevent and relieve stress.

Ailments practice chart

When planning your daily practice, refer to the chart on the opposite page. Each ailment in Part Three is listed here together with the postures, breathing exercises and meditation practices which you should focus on for each individual disorder. It also indicates which postures and breathing practices you should avoid if you have a particular condition.

KEY
Useful positions ●
Positions to avoid ✖

	NECK/SHOULDER STRETCHES	NECK ROLL	BACKWARD BEND	FORWARD BEND	SHOULDERSTAND	FISH POSE	BRIDGE POSE	CHILD POSE	HALF-HEADSTAND	DOG POSE	COBRA POSE	MOON POSE	LOCUST	CAT POSE	BOW POSE	SPINAL TWISTS	THE CORPSE	UJJAYI	NADI-SODHANA	SHITALI/SHITAKARI	CLEANSING BREATH	MEDITATION/RELAXATION	SUN SALUTATION	ABDOMINAL SUCTION
BACK PAIN				●		●					●		●	●		●		●				●		
VARICOSE VEINS					●	●														●				
NASAL ALLERGY																					●			
DIARRHOEA																●					●	●		
CONSTIPATION				●							●		●		●						●			
PMS											●				●	●					●	●		
MENSTRUAL PROBLEMS				●							●	●						●	●		●	●		
EPILEPSY			●		●									✖				●			✖			✖
HEART DISEASE												✖				✖	●	●	●			●		
HYPERTENSION	●							●	✖		●						●	●	●	●	✖	●	✖	✖
DIGESTIVE DISORDERS			●	●	●	●											●					●		●
DIABETES															●	●		●	●			●		
ASTHMA			●	●							●						●	●	●			●		
ARTHRITIS									✖															
HEADACHES		●			✖	✖				✖							●					●		
INSOMNIA	●																	●	●			●		
ANXIETY					●													●	●			●		
DEPRESSION							●		●	●									●		●	✖		
ADDICTION	●																				●	●		
PANIC ATTACKS					●												●	●	●					
ABDOMINAL HERNIA				✖												✖						●	✖	
COLDS																		●	●		●			
LUNG DISEASE																		●	●	●	●			
HYPERACIDITY																				●			●	
EYE PROBLEMS			●								●	●						●		●				
YOGA IN OLD AGE	●						●		●	●								●	●		●	●		
YOGA IN PREGNANCY	●																				✖	●		

HEART DISEASE

In the Western world, approximately half of all deaths are due to heart disease. There are many different types of condition which affect the heart and cardiovascular system, the commonest in developed countries being ischaemic heart disease.

When the blood supply to the heart wall is inadequate, nerve endings are stimulated, producing the gripping pain known as angina. It is easy to mistake angina for indigestion, as it is often felt around the mid-chest, sometimes deeply located. For this reason if you have any chest pain you should have it checked.

FACTORS CONTRIBUTING TO HEART DISEASE

Ischaemic heart disease is associated with smoking, obesity and a high intake of cholesterol and saturated fats. Some people may be at a greater risk due to genetic factors. There are many causes of ischaemic heart disease. It is an over-simplification to say that a stressful lifestyle alone leads to the condition. However, you may be able to reduce your risk of heart disease by avoiding smoking, and also by eating a healthy diet. If you lead a very active existence, you can cut down on your commitments, and slow down your pace. Also, you can make a conscious effort to relax by exercising regularly, or pursuing an enjoyable activity.

If you suffer from heart disease you can focus on the Corpse Pose (see p.52), Alternate-Nostril Breathing (see pp.53-4) and Victorious Breath (see p.55), and conclude with *Yoga Nidra* (see pp.114-17), and meditation (see pp.56-7; p.87; p.111). Do not hold the breath in any practice, and do not practise inverted postures without guidance.

CAUTION

If you are suffering from a heart condition, you should be under appropriate medical care. However, to complement the conventional treatment, you can consult a properly qualified yoga therapist.

ASANAS & PRANAYAMAS TO FOCUS ON:

The Corpse Pose
Alternate-Nostril Breathing
Victorious Breath
Deep Relaxation
Meditation

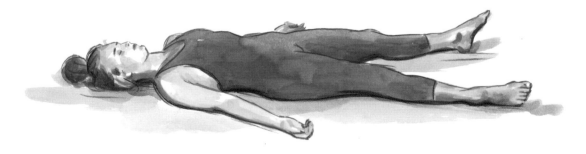

HYPERTENSION

The heart generates the pressure which drives the blood around the body. Thus "blood pressure" is an essential to life, and it is only when the pressure is too high or too low that a medical condition exists. In about 90% of cases no cause can be identified, and the condition is known as essential hypertension. Some of the causes of essential hypertension may include genetic makeup, overweight and excess alcohol consumption.

Hypertension can be brought on by long periods of over-stimulation, and has a strong emotional trigger. It frequently occurs when a person has constantly to adapt to changing emotional circumstances. Repeated stimulation of the hypothalamus results in "fight or flight" responses, including high blood pressure.

USING YOGA TO ALLEVIATE HYPERTENSION

By regular yoga practice, you can help to lower your blood pressure. If your hypertension is mild, you can practise the exercises below without supervision. If your condition is more serious, you can practise the meditations (see pp.56-7; p.87; p.111), the Corpse Pose (see p.52) and the Deep Relaxation (see pp.114-17), but you should not use any other physical exercises or breathing practices without the guidance of a qualified yoga therapist.

For mild hypertension, you can use the shoulder stretches and neck movements (see pp.40-51), followed by Alternate-Nostril Breathing (see pp.53-4) and Victorious Breath (see p.55) for ten minutes and conclude with twenty minutes relaxation in the Corpse Pose (see p.52). Do not hold the breath at any time in the breathing practices. Separately, you can practise the meditation on "peace" and "freedom" for twenty minutes (see pp.56-7).

In the following fortnight, you continue with the Moon Pose (see pp.96-7) or the Child Pose (see p.93), for a few minutes each, without holding the breath. Then add *Shitali* and *Shitakari* breathing practices (see p.86), for five minutes each. In the meditation session, combine the affirmations on contentment and the mental recitation. Alternate the latter with the repetition of a specific *mantra*, such as "Soham" ("I am one with the infinite spirit"), synchronising it with the breath inflow ("so") and outflow ("ham").

In the final weeks you can replace the Corpse Pose with the Deep Relaxation.

ASANAS & PRANAYAMAS TO FOCUS ON:
Shoulder stretches & neck movements
Alternate-Nostril Breathing
Victorious Breath
The Corpse Pose
The Moon Pose
The Child Pose
Shitali
Shitakari
Deep Relaxation
Meditation

DIGESTIVE DISORDERS

Most people suffer from indigestion at some time, and this is not usually at all serious, but regular bouts of heartburn, pain below the breastbone or vomiting may be signs of gastritis.

In peptic ulceration the lining of the stomach or of the duodenum breaks down, leaving a raw area. The precise cause of the ulceration is not clear.

Crohn's disease and ulcerative colitis are inflammatory bowel diseases. Crohn's disease affects any part of the small or large intestine, while ulcerative colitis is confined to the colon or rectum. Both disorders require long-term medical management.

Indigestion and irritable bowel syndrome (IBS) are both very common conditions in which psychological factors are of major importance. The symptoms are usually worsened by stress.

USING YOGA TO TREAT DIGESTIVE DISORDERS

If you have only a common disorder, such as IBS or constipation, you can practise yoga unsupervised, but if you suffer from any other condition you should only practise supervised by a therapist.

You can focus on the Shoulderstand (see pp.72-7) and the Fish Pose (see pp.78-9), followed by the Bridge Pose (see pp.82-4) and the Forward Bend (see p.85), combined with *Agnisara*, a good practice for digestive problems.

CAUTION

If you have peptic ulcers, Crohn's disease or ulcerative colitis you should be under the supervision of a yoga therapist. Do not practise the Shoulderstand, *Agnisara* or *Kapalabhari*.

ASANAS & PRANAYAMAS TO FOCUS ON:

The Shoulderstand
The Fish Pose
The Bridge Pose
The Forward Bend
Agnisara
Alternate-Nostril Breathing
Victorious Breath
Cleansing Breath
The Corpse Pose
Meditation

Follow the Shoulderstand series with the Alternate-Nostril Breathing (see pp.53-4) and Victorious Breath (see p.55), or Cleansing Breath (see p.110). You can conclude the session with the Corpse Pose (see p.52), or the Deep Relaxation (see pp.114-17), and the meditation practices, which will have a calming influence (see pp.56-7; p.87, p.111).

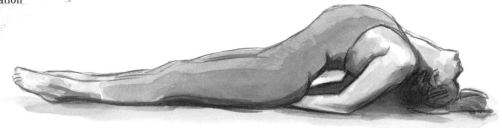

DIABETES

The commonest form of diabetes (*diabetes mellitus*) is a condition where too much sugar is present in the blood. It is vital that the brain, a major sugar consumer, is supplied with a constant supply of nutrition despite any irregularities of food intake or energy output. Blood sugar levels are controlled mainly by the hormone insulin secreted by the pancreas, although other hormones are also involved. There are two main types of *diabetes mellitus*, although there can be overlap between the two. Insulin-dependent *diabetes mellitus* (IDDM) is often diagnosed in middle childhood. IDDM is due to failure of the pancreas to produce enough insulin, so that treatment must include replacement therapy by regular self-injection, as well as dietary management.

Non-insulin-dependent *diabetes mellitus* (NIDDM) tends to be diagnosed in older people, and is more common in people who are very overweight. In NIDDM the insulin deficiency is only partial, but the body does not respond normally to the levels of hormone which are present (a condition known as insulin resistance). NIDDM is treated by diet and drug therapy, rather than insulin injection.

USING YOGA TO HELP MANAGE DIABETES

Although neither type of diabetes is caused by stress, many diabetics find that stress levels do affect their illness, both by influencing their appetite and therefore their food intake, and also by affecting the blood sugar levels directly.

If you have either IDDM or NIDDM you are more likely to develop other complications, such as kidney, retinal and cardiovascular disease, and both require long-term medical monitoring and careful management, especially in pregnancy.

If you have diabetes, you can practise any of the exercises in the Three-Month Programme, providing you adjust your food and/or insulin intake to allow for the increased physical activity. You can concentrate on the lumbar stretches from weeks three and four (see pp.60-9), the Shoulderstand (see pp.72-7), and the Cobra series (see pp.94-105), in particular the Bow (see pp.102-3). You should also practise the Simple-Spinal Twist (see p.104) and the Deep Relaxation (see pp.114-17). Regularly practise *pranayama* and build daily relaxation and meditation sessions into your routine.

ASANAS & PRANAYAMAS TO FOCUS ON
The Bow
The Simple-Spinal Twist
Deep Relaxation
Alternate-Nostril Breathing
Victorious Breath

HEADACHES

A headache is not a disease but a symptom which can be caused by many conditions, from the trivial to the life-threatening. The commonest type of headache, often referred to as a "tension" headache, is commonly attributed to muscle tension in the scalp or neck muscles; but this has not been scientifically proved. In general, "tension" headaches are not a sign of any serious underlying physical cause, and they are not a symptom of high blood pressure. They may be due to underlying depression or anxiety. Migraine headaches are often very severe and prolonged. They may be preceded by, or associated with, physical symptoms such as visual disturbance, tingling in the limbs and nausea. The visual disturbances can include temporary partial loss of vision, shimmering effects or the appearance of zigzag lines.

PHYSICAL FACTORS WHICH TRIGGER A HEADACHE

Sinusitis, or inflammation of the air–filled spaces in the skull bones, can be another cause of headaches. Sinusitis usually develops as a complication of an upper respiratory infection, and may require antibiotic treatment.

There are many other causes of headache, and if you feel worried, you should consult your doctor, especially if the headaches have started suddenly, or if they are associated with dizziness, weakness in the limbs or partial loss of vision that is not related to migraine.

If you suffer from chronic headaches or migraine, you can alleviate the problem by working through the Three-Month Programme, focusing upon relaxation techniques such as the Corpse Pose (see p.52), the Deep Relaxation (see pp.114-17) and the meditations (see pp.56-7; p.87; p.111). The Neck Roll (see p.51) is also very beneficial. You should avoid inverted postures like the Shoulderstand series (see pp.72-7), and head-down postures.

ASANAS & PRANAYAMAS TO FOCUS ON:
The Corpse Pose
Deep Relaxation
Meditation
The Neck Roll

INSOMNIA

Regular periods of sleep are essential for the body and mind to function properly. During a normal night's sleep, you experience periods of deep sleep associated with rapid eye movements and dreaming. People who suffer from insomnia find it difficult to fall asleep at night, or else wake intermittently through the night. They have insufficient periods of deep sleep and, instead of feeling refreshed in the morning, wake up feeling tired and irritable, and often remain so throughout the day. Chronic lack of sleep, for whatever reason, can lead to depression, muscle aches and pains and eventually complete collapse of normal functioning, both physical and intellectual.

There are many causes of insomnia. As we grow older our body naturally needs less sleep. Many elderly people find that around four or five hours per night is enough, and this cannot be said to be true insomnia. Young people on the whole sleep well, so therefore most people with sleep problems are young to middle-aged adults.

ASANAS & PRANAYAMAS TO FOCUS ON:
Shoulder stretches & neck movements
Deep Relaxation
Alternate-Nostril Breathing
Victorious Breath

THE POWER OF YOGA IN PROMOTING SLEEP

Insomnia is rarely a direct symptom of any serious disease, although sleeplessness can be due to a painful condition, such as arthritis. If you are depressed this can disturb your sleep patterns, and you may frequently wake early in the morning. For most people however, difficulty in sleeping well occurs at times when they have many worries on their mind, or when their body and mind are so stressed that they cannot relax into natural sleep. If you have insomnia you may be tempted to rely on sleeping tablets, and these may help you in the short term when prescribed by your doctor, but mostly they do not produce natural sleep with adequate periods of dreaming.

If you suffer from insomnia, you will find yoga of enormous benefit. The stretches in weeks one and two (see pp.40-51) are very beneficial if you practise them slowly. Avoid backward-bending movements in evening practice, as they raise energy levels. Yoga before bedtime will relax the body and quieten the mind, especially if you focus on Alternate-Nostril Breathing (see pp.53-4), Victorious Breath (see p.55) and the Deep Relaxation (see pp.114-17).

ANXIETY

Anxiety is the body's response to fear, and as such has a valuable role to play in self-preservation, its being the fear of the consequences which often prevents us from taking unnecessary risks. Anxiety as a disorder is an acute or chronic state resulting from the extent of the fear response becoming out of proportion to the actual risk. The body's response is at both a physical and mental level. Over-stimulation of the sympathetic nervous system leads to physical symptoms such as a racing heartbeat, sweating and trembling, while restlessness, insomnia and difficulty in concentrating are common psychological components.

If you are suffering from mild anxiety, you may only need some reassurance from your doctor, who will normally prescribe drug treatment only if your condition is acute. Yoga is invaluable in the management of anxiety, as its unique combination of gentle physical movements, breathing practices, relaxation and meditation are designed to harmonise the workings of the nervous system and to relax the physical body.

ASANAS & PRANAYAMAS TO FOCUS ON:
Victorious Breath
Alternate-Nostril Breathing
The Corpse Pose
The Shoulderstand

UNDERSTANDING AND MANAGING ANXIETY

Anxiety may be the result of temporary circumstances which you cannot change, for example the illness of a close relative, but if it is due to factors which lie within your sphere of influence, you should appraise your life and lifestyle, and look for ways to improve matters, so that you feel more in control. This will reduce your overall anxiety levels and allow you to cope more easily.

If you are suffering from anxiety, you can use all aspects of the Three-Month Programme. Before starting your practice, you should spend ten minutes in the Corpse Pose (see p.52). Use this time mentally to separate yourself from your experiences of the past, and from the anticipated happenings (real or imaginary) of the future. You should focus your awareness on the present moment only, and if your attention strays during the practice, quietly bring your mind back to this awareness. The relaxation induced by Alternate-Nostril Breathing (see pp.53-4), Victorious Breath (see p.55) and the Deep Relaxation (see pp.114-17), will quieten the mind, as well as resting the body.

DEPRESSION

Like anxiety, depression can be a temporary normal consequence of some of life's experiences, such as bereavement or redundancy. If, however, your negative mood persists for longer than usual, or deepens into an all-encompassing state, you may be suffering from a depressive condition and should seek professional help such as counselling or psychotherapy. It is important to find help if you are depressed, even if you do not think that it will do any good. Feelings of hopelessness are often part of the illness, and you may need to force yourself to ask your doctor for advice. Depression ranges from mild pessimism to overwhelming feelings of guilt, worthlessness and futility. If you are suffering from very severe depression you may feel suicidal, and should seek medical help without further delay.

OVERCOMING THE PHYSICAL SYMPTOMS OF DEPRESSION

The symptoms of mild depression include lack of energy, early morning wakening, appetite and weight loss. When you are depressed, you will usually feel very pessimistic and negative, but you may well respond, albeit temporarily, to changes in your environment such as an unexpected sunny day or a social event.

Severe depression usually requires hospitalisation, while mild to moderate depression can respond very well to yoga, especially if supervised by a yoga therapist trained in treating depressive disorders. If you are depressed, you can use all the exercises described in the Three-Month Programme. Back-bends, such as the lumbar stretch backward bend in weeks three and four (see p.60) and the Bridge Pose (see pp.82-4) are valuable, as they raise energy levels, and every morning you should practise the Sun Salutation (see pp.108-9) in weeks nine and ten, as this has an invigorating effect. In the summer it is particularly beneficial to perform *Surya-Namaskara* out of doors, providing you work out of the direct heat of the sun. You should resist the temptation to spend long periods of time in meditation, or in the Deep Relaxation (see pp.114-17), as this is not advisable if you suffer from depression – instead relax for shorter periods of time of not more than ten minutes.

ASANAS & PRANAYAMAS TO FOCUS ON:
The Bridge Pose
The Half-Headstand
The Dog Pose
Deep Relaxation
Meditation
Alternate-Nostril Breathing
Shitali
Shitakari
Cleansing Breath

ADDICTION

Addiction to a substance or a mode of behaviour can be indicative
of a particular personality type. The addict is usually lacking in
self-confidence and self-esteem, and initially makes use of the
addictive substance or behaviour because it helps to counteract
these feelings. Unfortunately, soon it becomes apparent to the
addict that this usage is no longer voluntary, and this realisation
only worsens the feelings of worthlessness and guilt.

Addiction can involve the overuse of a normally available
substance such as alcohol or cigarettes. Many people have become
addicted to prescribed medication, for example tranquillisers, while
others use illegal drugs or else misuse substances designed for other
purposes, such as solvents. Addictive behaviour is also very
common, for example in eating disorders. In *anorexia nervosa*,
the individual is addicted to not eating, while in *bulimia nervosa*
the sufferer eats large quantities of food and then vomits in secret.

Many people keep their addictions secret, and it is only when
they begin to have an effect on other people's lives that their
problem is discovered. The feelings of guilt are compounded by
this, and the addiction may then spiral out of control.

FINDING HELP FOR ADDICTION

If you have an addiction problem, it is important to realise that
help is at hand. Many treatment units and recovery programmes
are available, as well as self-help groups and specialist therapists.
While you are following a recovery programme, you can use
yoga to help your body and mind to relax. During the immediate
recovery period, construct an ordered daily routine, as this
will enable you to feel that you are now in control of your
life. Yoga should be given a regular place within that
routine, and you should work through the whole
programme steadily as described. Begin with the
opening shoulder stretches and neck movements
in weeks one and two (see pp.40-51). Practise the
postures more quickly than usual, pausing after
each group of *asanas* for three minutes of deep
breathing. The Deep Relaxation (see pp.114-17)
and *Kapalabhati* (see p.110) are also
particularly beneficial.

**ASANAS & PRANAYAMAS TO
FOCUS ON:**
Shoulder stretches & neck
movements
Deep relaxation
Cleansing Breath

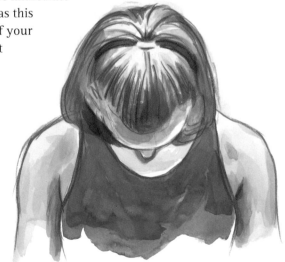

PANIC ATTACKS

A panic attack is an event in which the overactive sympathetic nervous system seems to run out of control. The symptoms can be very frightening – palpitations, sweating, dizziness, light-headedness and intense fear are all typical. A panic attack may come on for no apparent reason, or may be in response to exposure to some form of phobic stimulus such as feathers or spiders, or going out of doors in the case of someone suffering from agoraphobia.

Sufferers from panic attacks know that the episode is very frightening, but most fail to realise that fright is the cause, as well as the result. A sound understanding of what is happening in such an attack can help in its immediate treatment, and will also reduce the chances of its happening again. Some initial stimulus produces increased activity in the sympathetic nervous system, resulting in increased anxiety. The sufferer is then alarmed by this response, and their fearful anticipation of a rising tide of anxiety causes greater over-stimulation of the sympathetic nervous system. Thus the symptoms are redoubled, and the sufferer is in a short time in the grips of a full-blown panic attack. The breathing becomes shallow and so rapid that the sufferer hyperventilates. This indirectly disturbs the oxygen supply to the brain, so dizziness and light-headedness are experienced.

ASANAS & PRANAYAMAS TO FOCUS ON:
Victorious Breath
Alternate-Nostril Breathing
The Corpse Pose
The Shoulderstand

UNDERSTANDING AND MANAGING PANIC ATTACKS

The management and treatment of such an attack lies in the understanding that it is the fear which is causing the symptoms. "Riding out" the attack, by waiting quietly for it to pass, is a very helpful approach. Yoga can be invaluable both in helping you to manage the attack, and in reducing your underlying anxiety levels. You can control hyperventilation by using Victorious Breath (see p.55) or Alternate-Nostril Breathing (see pp.53-4). After an attack, if you are able, lie for several minutes in the Corpse Pose (see p.52) to allow your body to recuperate while the sympathetic nervous system activity returns to normal. Follow the Three-Month Programme, and practise the Shoulderstand sequence (see pp.72-7) slowly.

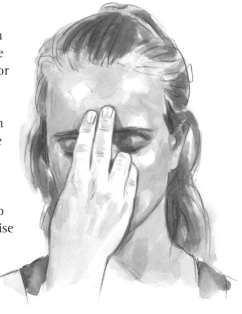

YOGA FOR THE ELDERLY

Yoga is probably of greater potential benefit to elderly people than to any other group. For maximum musculoskeletal health all the joints should be put through their full range of movement regularly, or they will start to stiffen. Weightbearing exercise, which loads the bones of the limbs and spine, will help to counteract the decline of bone density usually experienced in later life, particularly in post-menopausal women. This process can accelerate to produce osteoporosis, with subsequent fractures. Muscles also need regular work, or they will waste and become weakened.

As people age, they tend to give up the forms of exercise which they enjoyed in their youth, and become prey to stiffness, muscle weakness and general physical unfitness. Yoga postures and sequences work the muscles, which respond by becoming stronger. If you practise yoga daily, your joints will retain their suppleness, and it will be easier to manage osteoarthritis. The bones are loaded in weight-bearing postures, such as the Bridge Pose (see pp.82-4), the Half-Headstand (see pp.91-2) and the Dog Pose (see p.92).

THE BENEFITS OF YOGA IN LATER LIFE

If you are beginning yoga and are past middle age, you should attend a general class with an experienced teacher before attempting the Three-Month Programme, although the stretches in weeks one and two (see pp.40-51) should not present much problem and the breathing practices, meditations (see pp.56-7; p.87; p.111) and the Deep Relaxation (see pp.114-17) are all suitable.

Yoga is very beneficial for the frail elderly, although if you are very frail it is advisable to seek advice from a yoga therapist, who will be able to modify postures without losing their essence and benefit. If you are unable to work on the floor, you can adapt many postures for practice in a chair, or lying on a bed. You can raise your feet above your head against a wall when possible, and this is the only inverted pose you should attempt as an elderly beginner.

Frail and confused people often derive great pleasure and benefit from meditation and relaxation practices, which can be recorded on tape. Sleeping during these practices can be very beneficial as a form of deep relaxation, and should not be discouraged.

ASANAS & PRANAYAMAS TO FOCUS ON:
The Bridge Pose
The Half-Headstand
The Dog Pose
Shoulder stretches & neck movements
Alternate-Nostril Breathing
Victorious Breath
Cleansing Breath
Meditation
Deep Relaxation

YOGA IN PREGNANCY

Most women would like to approach pregnancy in the best possible health, both physical and mental. The birth itself is an intensely physical experience, for which the mother should try to prepare her body so that it is in peak condition. Mentally and emotionally, the time of waiting for the baby's arrival can be anxious and it will also be tiring, especially if there are other children to be cared for, plus job or other responsibilities. So yoga will be very beneficial during this time.

In early pregnancy, because of hormonal changes you may feel tiredness and experience intermittent nausea. At this time gentle yoga can be very beneficial, with emphasis on the stretches in weeks one and two (see pp.40-51), plus the Deep Relaxation (see pp.114-15). You should not practise the more demanding postures until the fourth month, and then only if your pregnancy is uncomplicated. As the baby grows you should omit postures which entail lying on your front, and any postures which become difficult on account of your changing body shape. During the middle three months you may very well experience an increased feeling of wellbeing, with your energy levels returning to pre-pregnancy values. At this stage you can use much of the Three-Month Programme, omitting the Shoulderstand and the prone postures, or any which are inappropriate on account of the "bump".

ASANAS & PRANAYAMAS TO FOCUS ON:
Shoulder stretches & neck movements
Deep Relaxation

RELIEVING PAIN AND DISCOMFORT IN PREGNANCY

Every pregnant woman will benefit from raising the feet above the heart for at least ten minutes daily. You can do this against the wall, and this will help to relieve the pressure of the womb against the pelvic veins, which can lead to varicose veins and swollen ankles at this stage of the pregnancy.

In the last three months of pregnancy you may experience low back pain due to the increasing weight of the womb. You should seek advice from a yoga therapist qualified to work with pregnant women. You can adapt standing forward stretches to accommodate the "bump", and on a regular daily basis you should raise your legs against the wall, and practise the Deep Relaxation (see pp.114-17). If you prepare for labour with the help of a yoga therapist, he or she will focus with you on standing and squatting postures, to strengthen your legs and loosen your hip joints.

RESOURCES

Finding a yoga teacher: To gain full benefits from your yoga practice you should find a teacher who will help you to learn the practices correctly. Most teachers of *Hatha* yoga will be familiar with the *asanas*, but only a few will be able to advise you on *pranayamas* and meditation practices. Standards of teaching vary dramatically, so it is worth taking time to find a good teacher. A personal recommendation is often the best way to find someone reliable. The organisations listed on pp.136–7 can provide you with information on classes in your area, lists of yoga organisations and developments in research. *Yoga and Health* magazine, which is published each month, has a comprehensive list of classes and courses held throughout the UK.

Yoga Biomedical Trust
PO Box 140
Cambridge CB4 3SY
Tel: 01223 367301
Fax: 01223 313587
Publish research material on use of yoga to treat and prevent specific illnesses and ailments.

Yoga Therapy Centre
Royal London Homoeopathic Hospital
60 Great Ormond Street
London WC1N 3HR
Tel: 0171 833 7267
Fax: 0171 833 7292
Information on yoga therapy and teacher training. Individual yoga therapy treatment for people with specific conditions such as asthma, back pain; group classes for specific conditions; general yoga classes; pregnancy and childbirth classes. Mail order goods – mats, books, video tapes and audio tapes.

Scottish Yoga Teachers Association
Frances Corr
26 Buckingham Terrace
Edinburgh EH4 3AE
Tel: 0131 343 3553
Registered teachers in Scotland; teacher training courses; seminars.

Yoga for Health Foundation
Ickwell Bury
Biggleswade
Bedfordshire SG18 9EF
Tel: 01767 627271
Yoga centre offering residential courses, weekly classes and training programmes.

Active Birth Centre
25 Bickerton Road
London N19 5JT
Tel: 0171 561 9006
Classes on yoga for pregnancy. List of teachers in UK trained to give classes in yoga for pregnancy.

Yoga and Health
21 Caburn Crescent
Lewes, E. Sussex BN7 1NR
Tel: 01273 473495
Monthly magazine. Lists classes, training courses and retreats throughout the UK.

Yoga Journal
2054 University Avenue
Berkeley
CA 94704
USA
Bimonthly magazine listing Hatha *yoga classes and training courses throughout the USA.*

Samata Yoga Center
c/o 4150 Tivoli Avenue
Los Angeles
CA 90066
USA
Tel: 001 213 306 8845
Fax: 001 213 306 4632
Supply information on yoga organisations in the United States.

Himalayan Institute of Yoga Science and Philosophy
RR 1, Box 400
Honesdale
PA 18431-9706
USA

Tel: 001 717 253 5551
Fax: 001 717 253 9078
Hatha *yoga and meditation courses. Residential programmes and meditation retreats.*

Yoga for Health Australia
Villa 6 - 14/16 Eddy Street
Thornleigh, NSW 2120
Tel: 00612 9875 1468
Offer Remedial Yoga Teachers Training Programme; workshops and seminars on Remedial yoga; introducing people with physical or mental problems to the healing aspects of yoga.

Yoga-Vedanta Academy
Shivananda nagar 249 192
Dist. Tehri-Garhwal, U.P.
Himalayas, India
Tel: 0091 135 430040
Fax: 0091 135 431190
Offers four two-monthly courses per year on Hatha *yoga, yoga philosophy and meditation.*

The Iyengar Institute
223A Randolph Avenue
London W9 1NL
Tel: 0171 624 3080
Classes in Iyengar yoga.

The Sivananda Yoga-Vedanta Centre
51 Felsham Road
Putney
London SW15 1AZ
Tel: 0181 780 0160

GLOSSARY

Adrenaline – hormone secreted by adrenal medulla in response to stress

Adrenals – endocrine glands on the top of each kidney

Agnisara – abdominal suction and stretch

Ardha-Matsyendrasana – Half-Spinal Twist

Ardha-Padmasana – Half-Lotus

Ardha-Sirshasana – Half-Headstand

Asana – posture

Ashram – a monastery

Bandha – muscular lock or contraction to control the flow of *prana*

Bhujangasana – Cobra Pose

Cardiovascular – relating to heart and blood vessels

Cerebral cortex – grey matter in the brain that covers the cerebrum

Dhanurasana – Bow pose

Endocrine gland – gland which secretes hormones into blood stream

Hatha yoga – practical branch of *Raja* yoga that includes the *asanas*, *pranayama*s and *kriyas*; "hatha" means sun and moon.

Hypertension – high blood pressure

Hypothalamus – nerve control centre at base of brain attached to the pituitary

Ida – one of the main *nadis*, flowing through the left nostril

Jalandhara-Bandha – chin lock

Kapalabhati – Breathing exercise which cleanses the respiratory system

Kriya – a purification practice

Matsyasana – Fish Pose

Meru-Vakrasana – Simple-Spinal Twist

Mudra – gesture or posture for controlling *prana*

Mula-Bandha – anal lock

Nadi – nerve channel in the energy body

Nadi-Sodhana – Alternate-nostril breathing

Neurone – cell specialised to conduct nerve impulses

Neurotransmitter – chemical by which a nerve cell communicates with another nerve cell or muscle

Pashimottanasana – Forward Bend

Pineal – pea-size gland in the brain that secretes melatonin into the blood stream

Pingala – one of the main *nadis*, flowing through the right nostril

Pituitary gland – principal endocrine gland regulating secretion in all other endocrine glands

Prana – vital energy or life force

Pranayama – regulation of breath; breathing exercise

Salabhasana – Locust

Sankalpas – intentions implanted in the subconscious in meditation

Sarvangasana – Shoulderstand

Setu Bandhasana – Bridge Pose

Shashankasana – Moon Pose

Shavasana – Corpse Pose

Shitakari – A body-cooling breathing exercise

Shitali – A body-cooling breathing exercise

Solar plexus – network of sympathetic nerves behind stomach that supply abdominal organs

Sukhasana – Easy Pose

Surya-Namaskara – Sun Salutation

Swanasana – Dog Pose

Thyroid – endocrine gland which secretes hormones that control metabolism and body growth

Uddiyana-Bandha – lock which raises diaphragm

Ujjayi – Victorious breath; breathing exercise

Vyaghrasana – Cat Pose

Yoga – Union of the individual soul with the Absolute

Yoga Nidra – deep relaxation or "yogic sleep"

FURTHER READING

Balaskas, Janet, **Preparing for Birth with Yoga**, Element, 1994.

Hewitt, James, **The Complete Yoga Book**, Rider, 1991.

Encyclopaedia of yoga practice including philosophy, history, meditation, asanas and pranayamas.

Iyengar, B K S, **Light on Yoga**, Aquarius Press, 1991.

Philosophy and practice of yoga. Postures and breathing exercises for beginners to advanced level.

Iyengar, B K S, **Illustrated Light on Yoga**, Thorsons, 1995.

Introduction for beginners to philosophy and practice of yoga. Practical programme suitable for beginners to intermediate level.

Iyengar, B K S, **Light on Pranayama**, Thorsons, 1995.

Practice programme of breathing techniques.

Mehta, Mira, **How to Use Yoga**, Lorenz Books, Anness Publishing, 1994.

Step-by-step guide to Iyengar method of yoga for relaxation, health and wellbeing.

Nagarathna, Dr R, Nagendra, Dr H R, Monro, Dr R, **Yoga for Common Ailments**, Gaia Books Ltd, UK, 1990.

Basic step-by-step yoga programme for maintaining health and fitness. Specific exercises tailored to treat common ailments.

O'Brien, Paddy, **Yoga for Women. Complete Mind and Body Fitness**, Thorsons, 1994.

Exercises to celebrate womanhood. Postures and breathing.

Stewart, Mary, **Yoga Over Fifty**, Little Brown and Company, 1995.

Step-by-step asanas – active and resting poses. Exercises for specific problems – insomnia, stiffness.

Weller, Stella, **Easy Pregnancy with Yoga**, Thorsons 1991.

Advice on nutrition, diet, stress management, stretching, breathing and relaxation techniques, regaining muscle tone and function after birth.

Weller, Stella, **The Yoga Back Book**, Thorsons, 1993.

Yoga exercises for people suffering from backache.

Weller, Stella, **Yoga for Children**, Thorsons, 1996.

Practical workbook of stretching and strengthening yoga exercises for children.

INDEX

AUTHOR'S ACKNOWLEDGEMENTS

The publication of this work would not have been possible without the initiative of Jane Sill, Editor of *Yoga and Health* magazine, and the interest of Pip Morgan, Managing Editor of Gaia Books. I wish to express my grateful thanks to both of them. It was Jane who took it upon herself to involve me in this project, and who offered to liaise with the publishers on my behalf. I wish to express my deep sense of gratitude to her.

I would also like to thank the students at the various yoga centres which I direct, and where I teach who helped me to devise a part of the Three-Month Programme. The shoulder and lumbar stretches in the first fortnight, and the variations on the traditional yogic postures were devised by myself with their co-operation.

My thanks are also due to various doctors working in various yoga centres who have advised me on how the specific yoga exercises in Part Three can help to alleviate stress-related physiological ailments.

In particular I would like to thank Dr K N Udupa, Emeritus Professor of the Institute of Medical Sciences of the Banaras Hindu University. I have drawn from his book, *Stress and its Management by Yoga*, in which he publishes his research into the psycho-physiological dynamics of stress. I have also referred to *A Systematic Course in Yoga and Kriya*, by my long-term former colleague, Swami Satyananda, at the Sivananda Ashram in Rishikesh, India.

With regard to the psychological aspects of stress, I have mainly drawn from my personal experience, and from the counselling work I have done with numerous people who have come to me with their stress-related problems over the past three and a half decades. Without taking into account their case histories, I could not have written Part One.

My thanks are also due to Clare Stewart, the Editor, to Jo Godfrey Wood, Editorial Supervisor, to Phil Gamble, Project Designer, and to all those involved in seeing through the publication of this work. Finally, my special thanks are due to Renate Gradenwitz, General Secretary of the Shivapremananda Foundation in Buenos Aires, for revising the written text.

PUBLISHER'S ACKNOWLEDGEMENTS

Gaia Books would like to thank the following for their help in the preparation of this book: Lynn Bresler, the proof-reader; Mary Warren for preparing the index; Desirée Kongerod of Tripsichore Yoga Theatre, Steven Mills and Lisa Boohan the models; the Tower Art Gallery and Local Museum Eastbourne for allowing us to use their site as a location for the photograph on p.112. The sculpture in the photograph is "Eighteen Thousand Tides", 1997, oak groynes weathered by the sea, by David Nash.